AF566977

INTERNATIONAL SERIES OF MONOGRAPHS IN
ORGANIC CHEMISTRY
GENERAL EDITORS: D. H. R. BARTON and R. A. RAPHAEL

VOLUME 9

THE TETRACYCLIC DITERPENES

THE TETRACYCLIC DITERPENES

J. R. HANSON

Lecturer in Chemistry,
University of Sussex

PERGAMON PRESS

OXFORD · LONDON · EDINBURGH · NEW YORK
TORONTO · SYDNEY · PARIS · BRAUNSCHWEIG

Pergamon Press Ltd., Headington Hill Hall, Oxford
4 & 5 Fitzroy Square, London W.1

Pergamon Press (Scotland) Ltd., 2 & 3 Teviot Place, Edinburgh 1

Pergamon Press Inc., 44–01 21st Street, Long Island City, New York 11101

Pergamon of Canada Ltd., 207 Queen's Quay West, Toronto 1

Pergamon Press (Aust.) Pty. Ltd., 19a Boundary Street, Rushcutters Bay, N.S.W. 2011, Australia

Pergamon Press S.A.R.L., 24 rue des Écoles, Paris 5e

Vieweg & Sohn GmbH, Burgplatz 1, Braunschweig

First edition 1968

Library of Congress Catalog Card No. 68–28684

PRINTED IN GREAT BRITAIN BY A. WHEATON & CO., EXETER

08 012550 6

CONTENTS

PREFACE

In this book I have tried to record the present status of a branch of natural product chemistry which has seen a rapid development over the last few years. The emphasis is primarily on recent studies which have served to clarify and unite some extremely interesting parts of terpenoid and alkaloid chemistry. This group of natural products, with a biological activity ranging from the plant-growth promoting properties of the gibberellins to the highly toxic aconite bases, has been the subject of study for more than a century. However, only within recent years have their structure and stereochemistry become known. Much of this is due to the powerful light that spectroscopic methods and X-ray analysis have shed on structural problems. It has been my good fortune to be able to witness some of this development over the last nine years.

I should like to record my thanks to my former colleagues at the Frythe, Drs. B. E. Cross, R. H. B. Galt, J. F. Grove, and J. MacMillan, for many interesting discussions. Professor D. H. R. Barton, F.R.S. suggested that I write this book and I am grateful to him for his encouragement and hospitality in enabling me to work at Imperial College. I am indebted to Miss Sue Wilson, who performed the difficult task of typing the manuscript. Finally a word of gratitude to Ann for her help and tolerance.

University of Sussex J. R. Hanson

CHAPTER 1

INTRODUCTION

THE diterpenes (or more accurately, the diterpenoids) form a widespread group of plant and fungal products derived from four units of isopentenyl pyrophosphate and thus containing about twenty carbon atoms. Their study has been pursued[1] throughout the long history of terpenoid natural product chemistry. However, for much of this time these efforts have been overshadowed by the investigation of the essential oils and by the study of the triterpenes and steroids. An explanation is not hard to find. Many of the earlier studies were confined to the resin acids. This proved to be an unhappy choice because of their ready isomerization and the consequent difficulties attending their purification. Indeed, prior to about 1920, that is for the first hundred years in the study of colophony, many experiments were performed with materials which are now known to have been impure. Furthermore, these compounds lacked the intrinsic biological interest of the steroids and the commercial value of the essential oils. However, within the last two decades a number of compounds of biological importance have been found amongst the diterpenes. Indeed it is now realized that they embrace a wide range of biological activity including antibiotics, plant hormones, cattle poisons and perfumery constituents.

The introduction of dehydrogenation experiments by Vesterberg[2] in 1903 and their subsequent exploitation[3] by Ruzicka and others during the inter-war years formed a major advance in terpenoid chemistry in the insight that its results shed on the underlying carbon skeleta of these polycyclic compounds. Coupled with the application[4] of the Biogenetic Isoprene Rule, again by Ruzicka, this provided the clarification of the major constituents of the plant resin acids. During the past two decades the widespread use of chromatographic methods of purification and the application of a variety of physical methods to natural product problems has had widespread repercussions. This is clearly seen in the rapid development of diterpene chemistry.

A number of classes of diterpene are now recognized which may be rationalized[4] as arising by cyclization of geranylgeraniol (I) possibly as its pyrophosphate (see Fig. 1). Although several schemes have been invoked to account for the various polycyclic skeleta, the major pathway

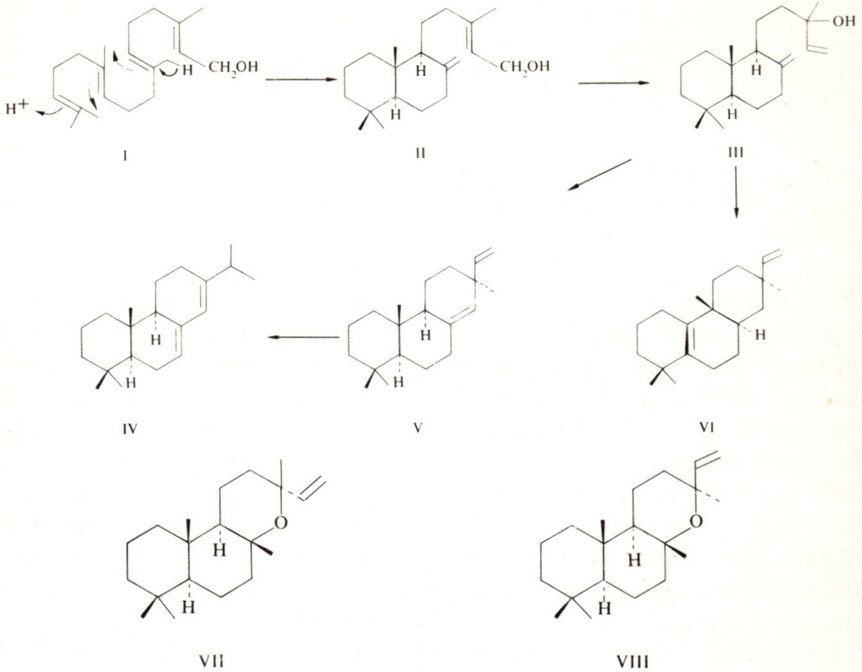

FIG 1.

appears to lead initially to the bicyclic diterpenes. These may be subdivided *inter alia* into those of the labdane (II) and manool (III) types. These included a number of resin constituents and a group of interesting bitter principles in which some subsidiary rearrangements have taken place. Cyclization of the bicyclic systems leads to the tricyclic abietadiene (IV), pimaradiene (V), and rosadiene (VI) skeleta, which form the backbone of many of the resin acids and their relatives. Further cyclization of the pimarane series then leads to the tetracyclic diterpenoids.

The tetracyclic diterpenoids, although quite widespread in nature, are structurally closely related. Indeed, they may be defined as diterpenoid natural products whose biogenesis lies through the cyclization of suitably oriented pimaradienes.[5] The bi- and tricyclic diterpenoids which are their biogenetic precursors, occur in two series epimeric at C-13 [e.g. manoyl oxide (VII) and 13-epimanoyl oxide (olearyl oxide) (VIII)]. Consequently cyclization of compounds of the (—)-pimaradiene (IX) and (—)-sandaracopimaradiene (XIII) series can lead to two different carbonium ion intermediates and hence to two distinct classes of tetracyclic diterpene differing in the relative disposition of ring D and the angular C-10 methyl group. This situation is further complicated by two features. Firstly, the fact that the carbonium ion intermediate may collapse in one of three ways, and secondly, that two *trans* A/B fusions occur—the normal (steroid-like) and the antipodal fusion. Thus cyclization of (—)-pimaradiene (IX) may produce compounds of either the (—)-kaurene (X), (+)-hibaene (stachene) (XI), or atisirene (XII) series whilst cyclization of (+)-sandaracopimaradiene (XIII) (related at C-13 to isopimaric acid) may lead to the phyllocladene series (XIV) and two hitherto unknown skeleta (cf. Ref. 6) the 8:13 isohibaene (XV) and 8:12 iso-atisirene (XVI). This is summarized in Fig. 2.

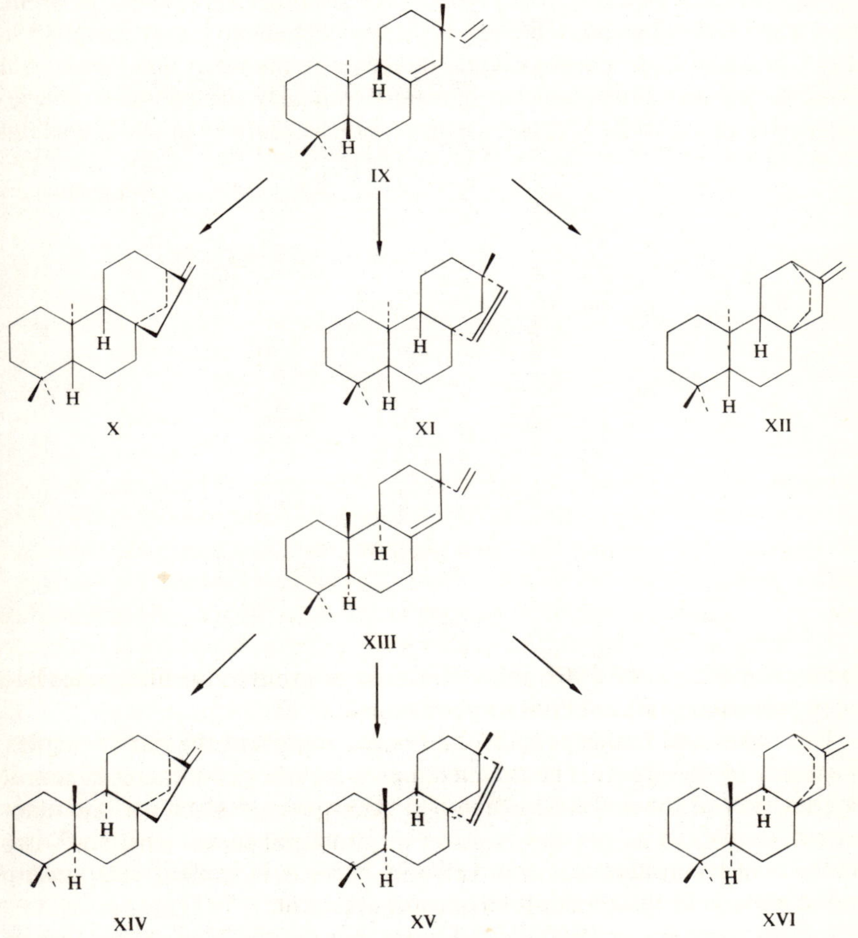

IX

X XI XII

XIII

XIV XV XVI

FIG. 2.

The distribution of compounds is such that the majority belong to the series derived from (—)-pimaradiene. Phyllocladene and phyllocladanol are at present the sole representatives of the other class. In view of their skeletal relationship to the tetracyclic diterpenes, the diterpene alkaloids of the Garrya (e.g. veatchine (XVII)), atisine and aconite classes will also be considered in this text. In these cases it would seem likely, but without experimental support, that the formation of the heterocyclic rings E and F represent a relatively late stage in the biosynthesis of these alkaloids.

Although phyllocladene was first isolated in 1910 from the leaf oil of *Phyllocladus rhomboidalis*, it remained the sole well-authenticated tetracyclic diterpene for many years. Its structure, proposed[7] in 1938, was not fully substantiated[8, 9] until its stereochemistry was assigned in 1959. Various hydrocarbons were described in the intervening years but their purity was often open to question. Similarly the complete stereochemistry of cafestol (XVIII), which was first isolated[10] in 1932, was not

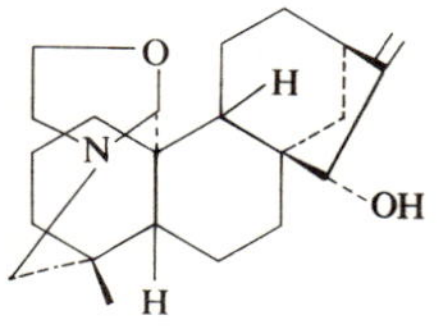

XVII

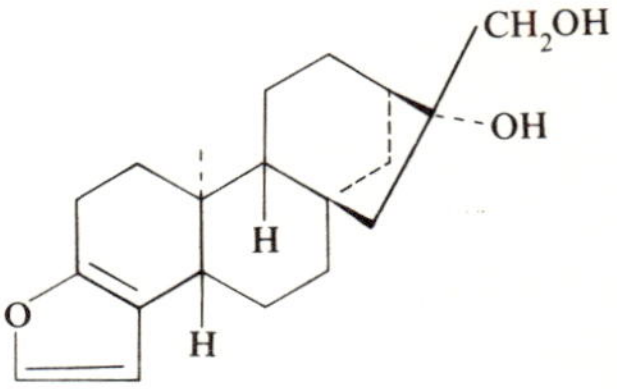

XVIII

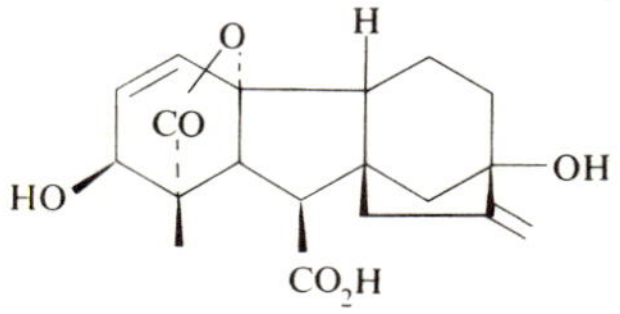

XIX

finally clarified[11] until 1962 although its relationship to the diterpenes had been proposed some twenty years previously.

The hexa- and heptacyclic aconite bases represent the most complex members of the group. The detailed and sometimes conflicting chemical degradation of these bases, which had been pursued since the late nineteenth century, was not rationalized in structural terms until an X-ray analysis of lycotonine was completed in 1956. A biogenetic relationship to the tetracyclic diterpenes then became apparent.

Indeed, whereas in 1956 the structure, but not the stereochemistry, of only a few compounds was known ten years later the full structure and stereochemistry of some eighty tetracyclic diterpenoids has been established. This rapid expansion is due to the widespread use of chromatographic techniques in separation and to the application of physical methods particularly nuclear magnetic resonance spectroscopy, in this branch of natural product chemistry. This is clearly exemplified by the study of the gibberellins. Initial work in this field was hampered by purification problems and although impure gibberellins were characterized[12] in 1938, the major chemical advances were not made until the late 1950's whilst the structure and stereochemistry of gibberellic acid itself (XIX) was not finally clarified[13,14] until 1962. Some twenty gibberellins have now been isolated whilst chromatographic evidence has indicated the presence of others.

The tetracyclic diterpenoids readily lend themselves to spectroscopic investigation. In marked contrast to the tetracyclic triterpenes, many of the functional groups occur on the pendant atoms of the carbon skeleton, as for example, primary alcohols and carboxylic acids. The routine application of nuclear magnetic resonance spectroscopy particularly favours this type of structural problem. Thus the determination of extra-skeletal methyl groups by the Kuhn–Roth procedure has been fraught with ambiguity in this series. Nuclear magnetic resonance methods readily provide an unambiguous answer. Olefinic unsaturation is confined mainly to ring D either as the terminal methylene of (—)-kaurene series or the cisoid double bond of the hibaene class. Here both infrared and nuclear magnetic resonance spectroscopy can provide valuable evidence for the presence of those functions. The development of optical rotatory dispersion and circular dichroism at a time when the stereochemistry of these skeleta was under investigation facilitated the solution of these problems. This evidence was particularly valuable in view of the occurrence of the antipodal A/B ring fusion and the differing types of ring D substitution.

The chemistry of the tetracyclic diterpenes is dominated by a number of features. Although the interpretation of many reactions rest upon analogies with steroid series there are some significant differences. Thus in view of the increased oxygenation on the pendant groups there are many examples of ether and lactone formation reactions. Furthermore, the transannular diaxial interactions, particularly those involving the angular methyl group, provide the driving force for a number of reactions and for skeletal distortions which find a closer analogy with the triterpenes than with the steroids. The control and knowledge of the stereochemical consequences of chemical reactions derived from experience in the syntheses of the steroids, is reflected in the several solutions to the total synthesis of the tetracyclic diterpenes which are now available.

With the interest in biosynthesis the close relationship of these compounds has led to the proposal[5,15] of a number of biogenetic schemes some of which have received experimental support. For example the presence of (—)-kaurene, the kaurenolides, and the gibberellins as fungal metabolites of *Gibberella fujikuroi* has provided[16] a ready means of testing some of these hypotheses.

In the first part of this text we shall describe the structural evidence for each of the classes of compound followed by a discussion of their synthesis and biosynthesis. The appendix comprises a catalogue of the known naturally-occurring tetracyclic diterpenes.

Nomenclature

Several schemes have been proposed for the numbering and naming of these compounds. In this text we shall follow that (XX)[17] which emphasizes the structural similarity between the di- and triterpenes. In numbering the geminal substituents at C-4 the equatorial substituent is numbered 18 and the axial substituent, 19. However, despite their relationship to the kauranoid class, we shall retain the gibbane (XXI) numbering[18] for the gibberellins in view of its now widespread acceptance

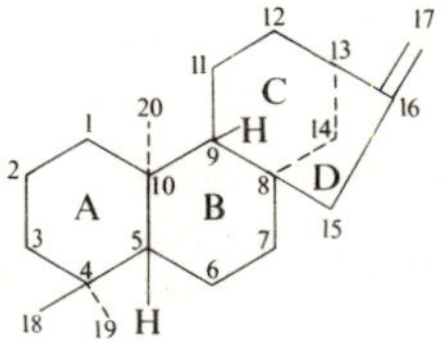

XX

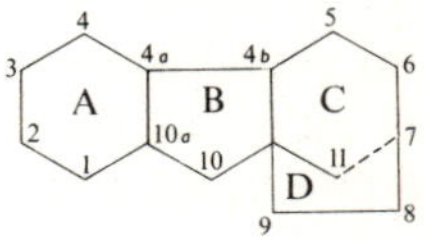

XXI

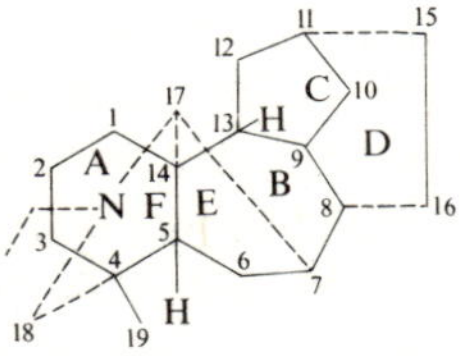

XXII

in the literature. For a similar reason the aconite bases are numbered as in (XXIV). Care should be taken in following this numbering as the geminal substituents at C-4 are numbered differently. The axial substituent is numbered 18 and the equatorial substituent, 19.

REFERENCES

1. Sir John Simonsen and D. H. R. Barton, *The Terpenes*, Vol. III, p. 328 *et seq.*, Cambridge University Press, London (1951).
2. A. Vesterberg, *Ber.*, **36**, 4200 (1903).
3. L. Ruzicka and L. Balas, *Helv. Chim. Acta*, **6**, 677 (1923).
4. L. Ruzicka, *Experientia*, **9**, 357 (1953); *Proc. Chem. Soc.*, 341 (1959).
5. E. Wenkert, *Chem. and Ind.*, 282 (1955).
6. E. Wenkert, P. W. Jeffs and J. R. Mahajan, *J. Amer. Chem. Soc.*, **86**, 2218 (1964).
7. C. W. Brandt, *N.Z. J. Sci. and Technol.*, **20**, 8B (1938).
8. L. H. Briggs, B. F. Cain, B. R. Davis and J. K. Wilmhurst, *Tetrahedron Letters*, no. 8, 8 (1959).

9. C. Djerassi, M. Cais and C. A. Mitscher, *J. Amer. Chem. Soc.*, **81**, 2386 (1959).
10. R. O. Bengis and R. J. Anderson, *J. Biol. Chem.*, **97**, 99 (1932).
11. A. I. Scott, G. A. Sim, G. Ferguson, D. W. Young and F. McCapra, *J. Amer. Chem. Soc.*, **84**, 3197 (1962).
12. T. Yabuta and Y. Sumiki, *J. Agric. Chem. Soc.* (Japan), **14**, 1526 (1938).
13. F. McCapra, A. I. Scott, G. A. Sim and D. W. Young, *Proc. Chem. Soc.*, 185 (1962).
14. D. C. Aldridge, J. F. Grove, R. N. Speake, B. K. Tidd and W. Klyne, *J. Chem. Soc.*, 143 (1963).
15. W. B. Whalley, *Tetrahedron*, **18**, 43 (1962).
16. B. E. Cross, R. H. B. Galt and J. R. Hanson, *J. Chem. Soc.*, 295 (1964).
17. L. H. Briggs, B. F. Cain, R. C. Cambie and B. R. Davis, *J. Chem. Soc.*, 1840 (1962).
18. J. F. Grove, *Quart. Rev.*, **15**, 56 (1961).

CHAPTER 2

THE KAURENE-PHYLLOCLADENE CLASS

THE members of the kaurene-phyllocladene class of diterpenes form the best known and most widely distributed of the tetracyclic diterpenes. Although phyllocladene was the first tetracyclic diterpene to be isolated and to have its structure determined, together with phyllocladanol, it remains the sole example to date of the trans-*anti*-trans backbone in this series. The majority of compounds in this group have the trans-*anti*-cis backbone and antipodal A/B ring fusion of (−)-kaurene. This is now not unexpected in view of the implication of (−)-kaurene in the biosynthesis of the gibberellin plant growth hormones. In this chapter we shall present firstly the evidence for the structure and stereochemistry of phyllocladene and then that of the kauranoid group of diterpenes.

2.1. *Phyllocladene*

Since its first isolation[1] in 1910 from *Phyllocladus rhomboidalis*, phyllocladene (I) has been found in a number of *Podocarpaceae*. A taxonomic survey[2] of the distribution of diterpene hydrocarbons utilizing gas–liquid chromatography demonstrated its presence in the essential oils of *Podocarpus dacrydioides*,[3,4,5] *P. henckelii*, *P. macrophyllus*,[6,7] *P. alpinus*, *P. hallii*, *P. nivalis*,[8] *P. nubigenus*, *P. andinus*, *P. ferrugineus*,[9,10] *P. montanus*, *P. spicatus*,[11] *P. totara*,[8(cf. 2)] *Dacrydium bidwellii*, *D. colensoi*, [12,13] *D. cupressinum*, [13,14,15] *D. franklini*, *D. biforme*, [16,17] *D. kirkii*,[18] and *D. laxifolium*, *Phyllocladus alpinus*,[13,19,20] *P. glaucus*,[21] *P. trichomanoides*.[22] *Araucaria excelsa*,[13,23,24] *Cupressus macrocarpa*,[25] and *Libocedrus plumosa*. Phyllocladene is identical to dacrene[16] (from *Dacrydium colensoi*), to sciadopitene[27] (from *Sciadopitys verticillata*) and iosene[28] isolated from various lignites. Mirene is a mixture of phyllocladene and (+)-kaurene.[2]

Phyllocladene was characterized[13] as a mono-unsaturated hydrocarbon by the formation of epimeric α- and β-dihydroderivatives, a hydrochloride and a dibromide. The carbon skeleton was partially identified by dehydrogenation[20,30] to pimanthrene (II) and retene (III). The position of the fourth ring and the double bond on this backbone was established by spectral investigation[31] and oxidative degradation.[30] Oxidation with neutral potassium permanganate gave the corresponding 16,17-diol,

17-norphyllocladan-16-one and the keto-acid (IV). The diol formed[32] both a 17-mono- and a diacetate whilst on benzoylation it gave a dibenzoate and under more vigorous conditions the unsaturated 17-benzoate.

One point of fusion of this cyclopentane ring was revealed[30] by reacting the ketone (IV) with methyl magnesium iodide, followed by dehydrogenation to give pimanthrene (II). The nature of ring D was further confirmed[31] by the infrared spectrum which showed that the norketone derived from phyllocladene was present in a five-membered ring and that there was only one methylene adjacent to the carbonyl group.

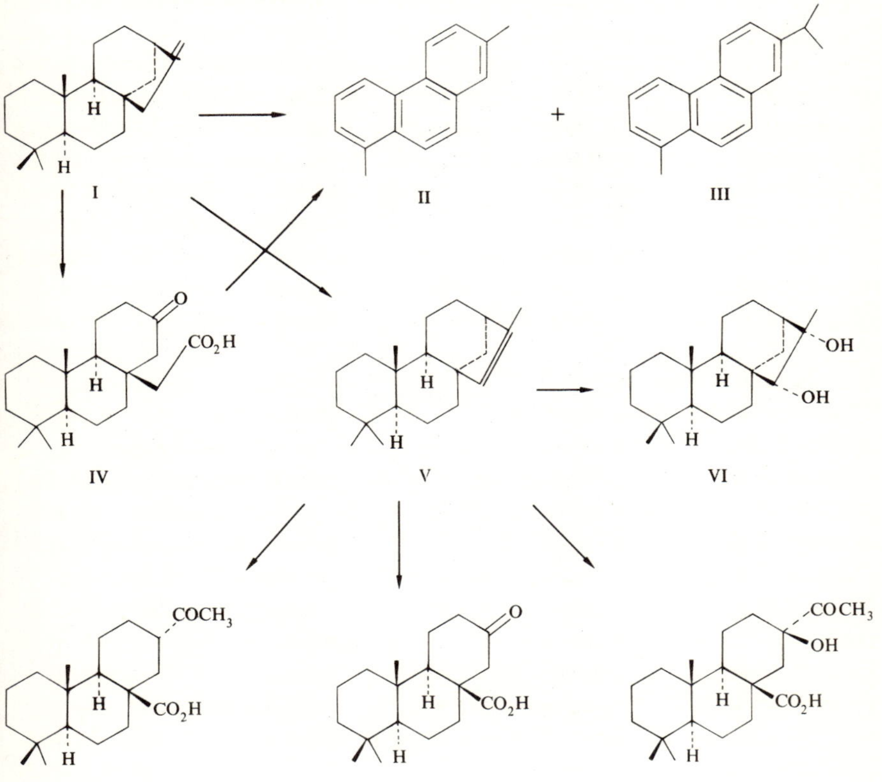

H H I + II III

CO_2H H H IV H H V OH OH H H VI

$COCH_3$ H CO_2H H VII O H CO_2H H VIII $COCH_3$ OH H CO_2H H IX

Acid-catalysed isomerization of phyllocladene gave isophyllocladene (V).[27,32–34] The products of oxidation of isophyllocladene with potassium permanganate are dependent upon the reaction conditions.[32] Thus aqueous potassium permanganate gave the diol (VI) and the keto-acid (VII). Under anhydrous conditions some allylic hydroxylation apparently takes place. The acidic products comprised the keto-acids (VII), (VIII) and (IX). Treatment of isophyllocladene with osmium tetraoxide gave the diol (VI).[30,35] On oxidation of this diol with chromium trioxide in pyridine or chromic acid–sulphuric acid, the $\alpha\beta$-unsaturated ketone (XI) formed the major product.[35] Cleavage of the diol with lead tetra-acetate[35] or sodium periodate[32] gave the keto-aldehyde (X) which was readily cyclized to the $\alpha\beta$-unsaturated ketone. The keto-aldehyde (X) was epimerized by alkali to the more stable α-isomer (XII). Further oxidation of the aldehyde (XII) with chromium trioxide in acetic acid gave the keto-acid. This underwent Baeyer–Villiger oxidation, hydrolysis to a hydroxy-acid, and further oxidation to form the bisnorketo-acid (VIII). Reduction of the keto-acid (VIII) with sodium borohydride led to ready formation of the lactone (XIII).

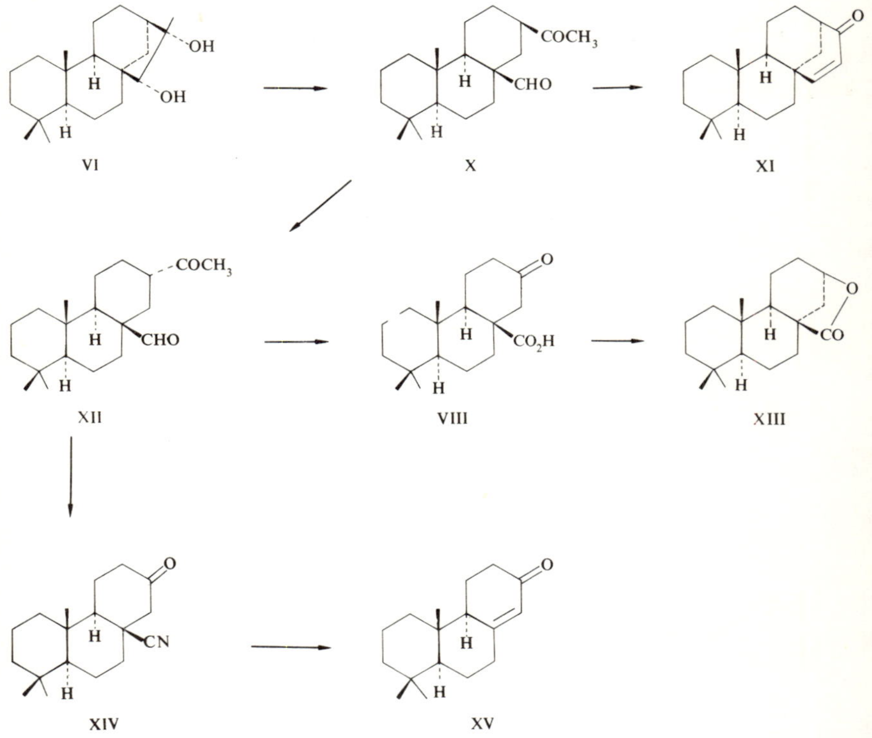

VI X XI

XII VIII XIII

XIV XV

The evidence for the stereochemistry of phyllocladene may be summarized as follows. Degradation of (+)-isophyllocladene to podocarp-8(14)-en-7-one (XV) established the "normal" nature of the A/B fusion and the position of the pendant methyl groups. This unsaturated ketone is a degradation product[36] of manool and is of known stereochemistry[37] whilst its racemate has been synthesized.[38–41] The dioxime of the keto-aldehyde (XII) on dehydration with acetic anhydride, gave a keto-nitrile which was subjected to Baeyer–Villiger oxidation, hydrolysis, and further oxidation to give the cyano-ketone (XIV). Elimination of hydrogen cyanide then gave the required $\alpha\beta$-unsaturated ketone (XV). Since the optical rotatory dispersion curve[34,42] of (+)-17-norphyllocladan-16-one and the ester of the acid (VIII) showed positive Cotton effects, ring D was assigned a β absolute configuration. This established the structure and stereochemistry (I) for (+)-phyllocladene.

A direct correlation[43] between (+)-phyllocladene (I) and (—)-kaurene (XVII) provided evidence for the stereochemistry of the latter. Baeyer–Villiger oxidation of 17-norphyllocladan-16-one formed a δ-lactone which was hydrolysed, methylated and oxidized to the keto-ester (XVI). The optical antipode of this keto-ester was prepared[44] from (—)-kaurene by opening ring D as a δ-lactone. Since the corresponding hydroxy-acid could not be obtained pure by hydrolysis of the lactone, the latter was reduced with lithium aluminium hydride to a diol which on oxidation afforded, *inter alia*, the lactonol (XVIII). Treatment of this lactonol with

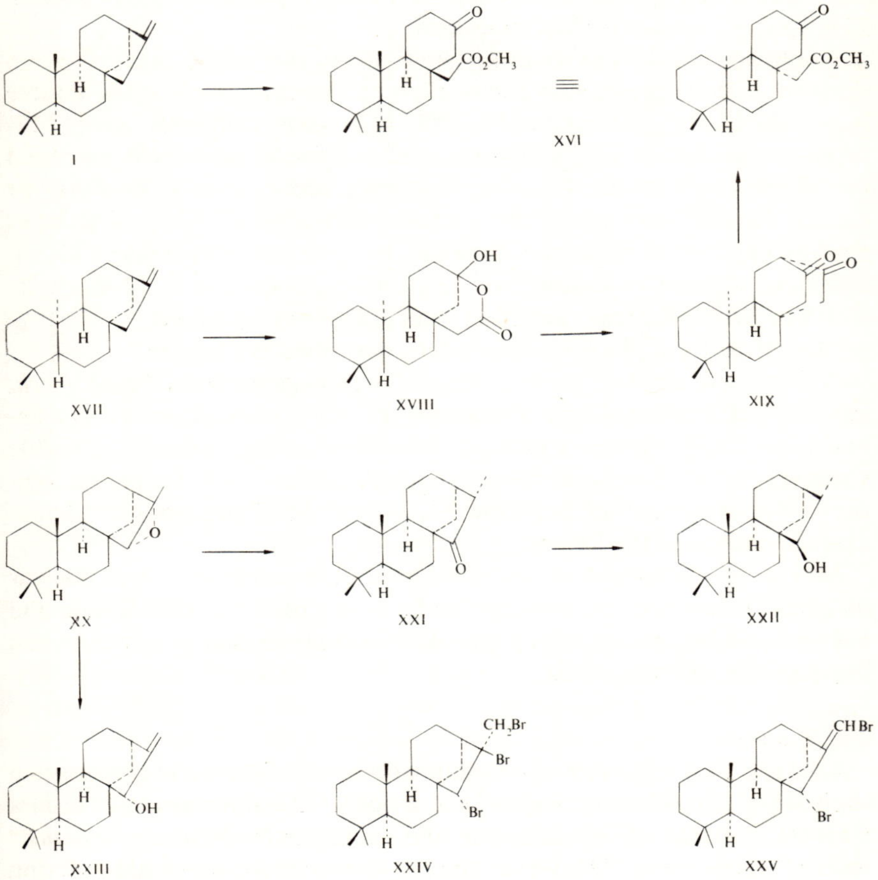

I → XVI ≡ XVI

XVII → XVIII → XIX → XVI

XX → XXI → XXII

XX → XXIII

XXIV

XXV

sodium methoxide and methyl iodide gave the required methyl ester. During this reaction inversion at position 8 had taken place by way of an intramolecular Claisen condensation at C-12 followed by fission of the resultant 1:3-diketone (XIX).

Two 15-ketones were derived from isophyllocladene by rearrangement[45] of the 15,16-epoxide (XX) with boron trifluoride etherate or magnesium bromide. Their stereochemistry was assigned on the basis of the amplitude of the Cotton effects in their optical rotatory dispersion curves and their relative stability to alkali. Reduction of the more stable 16-epiphyllocladan-15-one (XXI) with sodium borohydride gave 16-epiphyllocladan-15β-ol (XXII) as the major product in which attack of the hydride ion took place from the less hindered face of the molecule.

Reduction[46] of 15,16-epoxyphyllocladene (XX) with lithium aluminium hydride gave phylloclad-16-en-15α-ol (XXIII) as the major product together with some phyllocladan-16α-ol. The former was identical with the product of vigorous benzoylation (and dehydration) of phyllocladan-15α, 16-diol followed by saponification.

Isophyllocladene was hydroxylated[47,48] at the allylic methyl group during the Prévost reaction rather than by direct addition to the double bond. Similarly bromination[29] with N-bromosuccinimide gives 17-bromophylloclad-15-ene, whilst even the addition of bromine is preceded by allylic bromination, bromine in glacial acetic acid, chloroform or carbon tetrachloride giving the tribromo-derivative (XXIV). The latter readily eliminated hydrogen bromide to give the dibromide (XXV). Selenium dioxide oxidation[48] of isophyllocladene gave a 17-aldehyde which on Wolff–Kishner reduction regenerated phyllocladene.

The synthesis of phyllocladene will be described in Chapter 7.

A saturated alcohol, phyllocladanol[49] was isolated from *Cryptomeria japonica*. It contained one unreactive tertiary hydroxyl group. On dehydration the alcohol gave phyllocladene thus leading to the two possible structures of phyllocladan-16-ol and phyllocladan-17-ol. Its partial synthesis by reduction[46] of both the 15,16- and 16,17-epoxides of phyllocladene confirmed the former.

Mirene has been shown[2] by gas–liquid chromatography and nuclear magnetic resonance spectroscopy to be a mixture of phyllocladene and kaurene and hence the various speculative discussions of its structure and biosynthesis will be ignored.

2.2. *Kaurene*

Kaurene (XXVI) occurs in both enantiomeric forms and possesses a skeleton of considerable importance amongst the diterpenes. It occurs with the "normal" A/B ring fusion (the + form) in *Podocarpus spicatus*[50] and in *P. ferrugineus*.[10] However, the (–)-form with the antipodal A/B ring junction has been isolated from *P. macrophyllus*[6,7] and, surprisingly, from *Agathis australis*,[7,51,52] the source of a bicyclic diterpene, agathic acid, which possesses the normal A/B fusion. (—)-Kaurene also occurs in the mould *Gibberella fujikuroi*[53] along with the gibberellins. Its implementation[54] in the biosynthesis of the latter suggests a much wider occurrence. Amongst the Podocarpaceae, it has been detected[2] in *Podocarpus latifolius*, *P. nivalis*, *P. nagi*, *P. andinus*, *Dacrydium franklini*, *Phyllocladus trichomanoides*, *Araucuria auracana*, *Cupressus macrocarpa*, and *Sciadopitys verticillata*.[33] The α-podocarprene of the earlier literature[6] is identical[7,52] with kaurene whilst δ-podocarprene[6] and α-cryptomerene from *Cryptomeria japonica*[55] are identical with isokaurene, an acid-catalysed isomerization product comparable with isophyllocladene.

On selenium dehydrogenation[51,56] kaurene gave both pimanthrene and retene, isolated as their quinones. Hydrogenation of the one double bond gave α-[7] and β-dihydrokaurene (kaurane and 16-epikaurane) in which the former predominated, whilst hydrogenation of isokaurene gave almost entirely α-dihydrokaurene. Ozonolysis of the double bond gave formaldehyde and a cyclopentanone (XXVII) (ν_{max} 1745 cm^{-1}) and hence it formed the exocyclic methylene typical of the series. Infrared (ν_{max} 876 cm^{-1}) and nuclear magnetic resonance spectra (τ 5·27) confirmed these results. They also indicated that the double bond of isokaurene was trisubstituted (ν_{max} 820 cm^{-1}, τ 4·93).

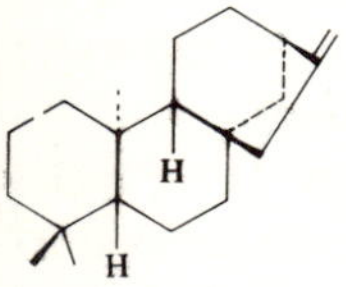

XXVI

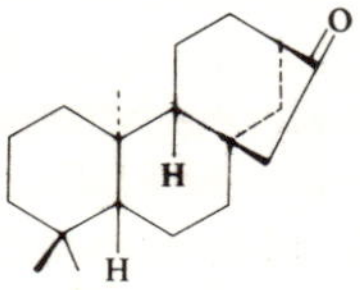

XXVII

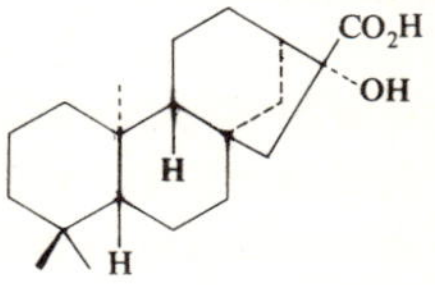

XXVIII

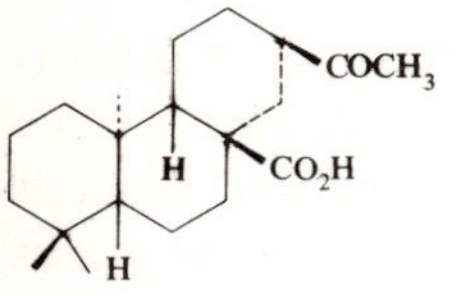

XXIX

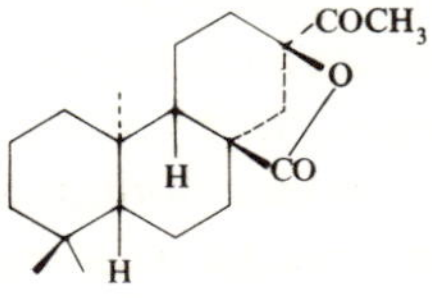

XXX

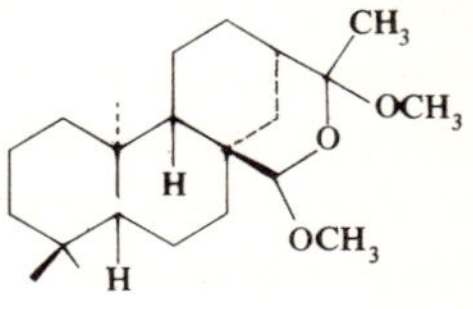

XXXI

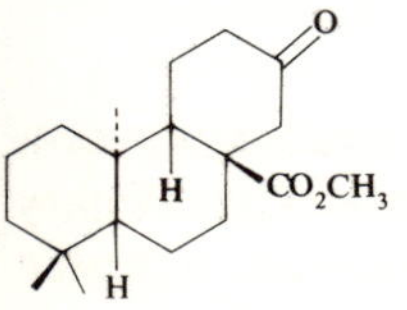

XXXII

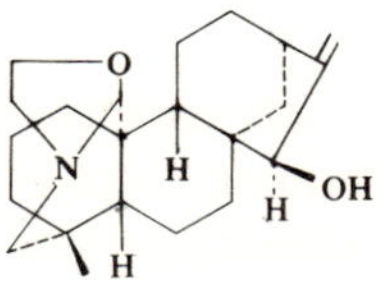

XXXIII

Oxidation and dehydrogenation of both kaurene and isokaurene gave results paralleling the phyllocladene series and leading to the overall structure (XXVI) for (–)-kaurene. Thus oxidation of kaurene with potassium permanganate gave the norketone (XXVII) and a hydroxy-acid (XXVIII) whose structure was confirmed[44] by cleavage with sodium periodate or sodium bismuthate[56] to the norketone. Reaction with osmium tetraoxide gave a 16,17-diol which was further converted to the norketone by treatment with lead tetraacetate or sodium periodate. Oxidation of isokaurene with dry potassium permanganate afforded kaurene 15α, 16-diol, 16-hydroxykauran-15-one and a keto-acid (XXIX). Use of osmium tetraoxide formed the 15,16-diol or with t-butyl hydroperoxide at 50°, the α-ketol. Oxidation of the ketol with periodic acid led to the γ-lactone (XXX) which was unchanged by further treatment with chromium trioxide. Oxidation of the diol with lead tetraacetate and crystallization of the oily keto-aldehyde from methanol led to the methoxy-ketal (XXXI). Baeyer–Villiger oxidation of the keto-acid (XXIX) followed by saponification, methylation and oxidation, gave a keto-ester (XXXII) utilized for rotatory dispersion measurements.

The evidence for the stereochemistry of (–)-kaurene rests upon the conversion of 7-hydroxykaurenolide,[57] steviol[58,59] and the diterpene alkaloid garryfoline[60,61] (XXXIII) to (–)-α- and β-dihydrokaurene. These degradations together with the correlation[43] with (+)-phyllocladene led, after some dispute, to a mutally consistent absolute configuration. In confirmation of this kaurene has been synthesized (see Chapter 7).

2.3. *The Kaurenolides and the Stereochemistry of (–)-Kaurene*

Although the gibberellins are well-known metabolites of the fungus *Gibberella fujikuroi*, the mould also elaborates a further group of diterpenoid metabolites which, whilst lacking the intrinsic biological interest of the gibberellins, have nevertheless taken their place amongst the expanding group of tetracyclic diterpenes. The major kaurenolides,[53,57] 7-hydroxy- and 7,18-dihydroxykaurenolide, (XXXIV) and (XXXVI) were characterized[62,63] through their derivatives and spectral properties as mono- and dihydroxy-γ-lactones containing one double bond present (from infrared and ozonolysis studies) as an exocyclic methylene group on a five-membered ring. The isolation[53] of the known natural products, (–)-kaurene and (–)-kauranol, from the culture filtrate implied a relationship with these metabolites which was subsequently established experimentally.

The inter-relationship of the metabolites, in which 7-hydroxykaurenolide formed the key intermediate, was achieved as follows. The primary hydroxyl group of 7,18-dihydroxykaurenolide was selectively acylated with toluene-p-sulphonyl chloride. This monotoluene-p-sulphonate on reduction with lithium aluminium hydride, gave a triol (XXXV) which was also obtained by reduction of 7-hydroxykaurenolide. A minor metabolite, 7β,16,18-trihydroxykaurenolide, can be obtained from 7,18-dihydroxy-kaurenolide by the action of mineral acid.

7-Hydroxykaurenolide was reduced[62] to (–)-kaurane (XXXIX) through a reaction sequence which precluded epimerization at any of the ring junctions. The epimeric 16-dihydro compounds were separated and the 6-oxygen function eliminated by hydrogenolysis of the 7-keto-lactone (XXXVII) with zinc dust. The 7-ketone was subsequently removed through a Wolff–Kishner reduction and then the 19-carboxyl converted to a methyl group by reduction of the methyl ester with lithium aluminium hydride to the alcohol (XXXVIII). The degradation was completed by oxidation of this to its corresponding aldehyde and finally Wolff–Kishner reduction. This degradation at the same time formed a link with steviol and the garryfoline alkaloids since the intermediate alcohol (XXXVIII) was formed in the degradation of those compounds to the hydrocarbon.

Implicit in this degradation was the presence of an acylated α -glycol on ring B including a $19 \rightarrow 6\alpha$-γ-lactone. 7-Hydroxykaurenolide was oxidized to a cyclohexanone, the presence of which was substantiated by the conversion of the dicarboxylic acid(XLI) through an unstrained adipic anhydride to a cyclopentanone. Hydrolysis of the kaurenolide led to an α-glycol. On oxidation, this gave a diketone which enolized to a diosphenol (XL) whose ultraviolet spectrum (λ_{max} 281 mμ) required a fully substituted chromophore – possible only on rings B or C. Oxidation of the diosphenol led to the formation of the dicarboxylic acid (XLI) which did not behave as a β-keto-acid – a situation which might have been expected had ring C been cleaved. Elimination of the 7-tosyloxy group from the toluene-*p*-sulphonate of 7-hydroxykaurenolide produced an enol-lactone (XLII) which was sterically possible only with the enol in ring B and the lactone carbonyl at the geminal position.

The nuclear magnetic resonance spectrum of 7,18-dihydroxykaurenolide showed that it contained only one *C*-methyl group and that a primary alcohol replaced the second methyl group of 7-hydroxykaurenolide. Two facets of its chemistry – namely the thermal loss of formaldehyde by a retroaldol reaction and the oxidative decarboxylation of the primary alcohol – indicated that the geminal methyl groups of (–)-kaurene both bore oxygen substituents in 7,18-dihydroxykaurenolide.

The stereochemistry of the kaurenolides and hence that of (–)-kaurene (which was open to doubt at the time of this work) involved a number of pieces of evidence. At C-4 it was possible to distinguish between the axial carbonyl of the lactone ring and the equatorial hydroxymethyl substituent by the hydrogenolysis of the less hindered 18-toluene-*p*-sulphonate as opposed to hydrolysis of the 19-toluene-*p*-sulphonate on

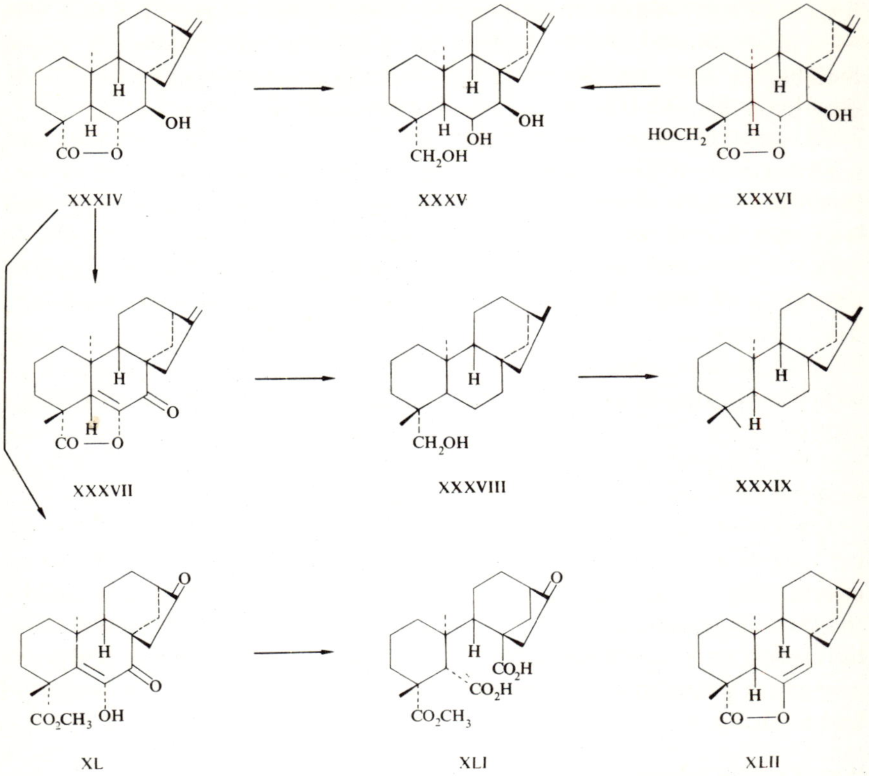

XXXIV XXXV XXXVI

XXXVII XXXVIII XXXIX

XL XLI XLII

treatment with lithium aluminium hydride and by pK^*_{MCS} measurements of the derived acids.[cf. 64] The *trans* diaxial relationship of the oxygen atoms on ring B was demonstrated in a number of ways. Reduction of the 7-ketones with sodium borohydride led to 7-alcohols epimeric at this centre with the natural alcohols. Comparison of the relative rates of elimination of the 7-toluene-*p*-sulphonates showed little difference between the epimers and hence there was no *trans*-diaxial relationship between a hydrogen atom at C-6 and the leaving group. Furthermore, whereas hydrolysis of the natural kaurenolides gave the corresponding 6,7-diols in high yield, hydrolysis of their 7-epimers gave along with the diols, a 25–30 per cent yield of the 6-deoxy-7-ketones by the diaxial elimination of water. The natural diols were inert to oxidation with sodium periodate whilst their 7-epimers reacted rapidly. Hence in the kaurenolides there is a *trans* relationship between the 6 and 7 oxygen substituents.

The presence of a 19 → 6 diaxial lactone ring precluded the existence of a *cis* A/B ring junction. Furthermore, oxidation of the 7-epihydroxy-19-lactone with lead tetraacetate led to the formation of a 7–20 ether thus demonstrating a *cis*-relationship between the hydroxyl group and the angular methyl group. Therefore the relative stereochemistry of the oxygen functions and the angular methyl group required the presence of the fragment (XLIII) in 7-hydroxy and 7,18-dihydroxykaurenolides. Since methyl 7-oxo-(−)-kauran-19-oate (XLIV) showed a large positive Cotton effect in its optical rotatory dispersion curve whilst the corresponding lactone showed a negative effect superimposed on a positive background, the lactone ring on formation must close axially into a negative quadrant and thus (XLIII) represents the absolute stereochemistry of rings A and B. The 16-ketones showed positive Cotton

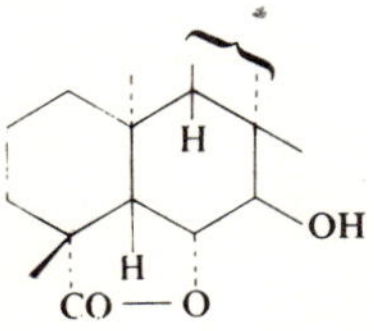

XLIII

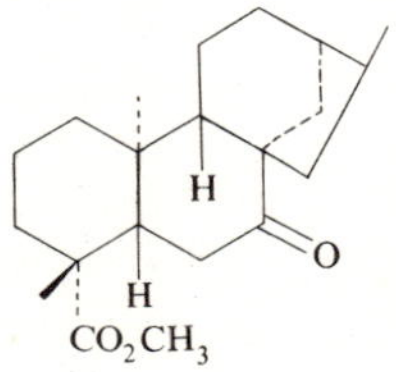

XLIV

effects and hence ring D possessed a β-absolute configuration. Thus the overall stereochemistry of (−)-kaurene and the kaurenolides must be represented by (XXVI), (XXXIV), and (XXXVI) respectively, in agreement with deductions drawn from studies with steviol and the garryfoline alkaloids.

2.4. *The Chemistry of Ring B of the Kaurenolides*

A more detailed examination[65] of the nuclear magnetic resonance spectra of the kaurenolides suggests that ring B exists in a twisted boat form bringing the 7-epihydroxy group into close proximity to the angular methyl group. Chemical evidence for this stems from the photochemical activation of C-20 from this position. Thus irradiation of the alcohol (XLV) in the presence of iodine and lead tetraacetate led to the formation of a 7–20 ether (XLVI). Ring B was shown to remain intact by reduction of the lactone to a diol and the subsequent reoxidation of this to a lactonol. In the latter the C-7 proton then collapsed to a singlet.

Treatment of the 7-equatorial toluene-*p*-sulphonate (XLVII) with base led[66] primarily to hydrolysis of the lactone and the formation of (XLVIII). However, a minor product (XLIX) possessed the gibbane skeleton. This not only formed a link with the gibbane series but also provided[67] part of the evidence for the structure of gibberellin A_{12}. A 7-axial epimer under similar conditions gave the $6\alpha,7\alpha$-epoxide (LI).

The elimination reactions of the 7-epimeric alcohols were used to define the conformation of ring B. Treatment of both 7-epimeric toluene-*p*-sulphonates with lithium iodide in collidine led to the formation of

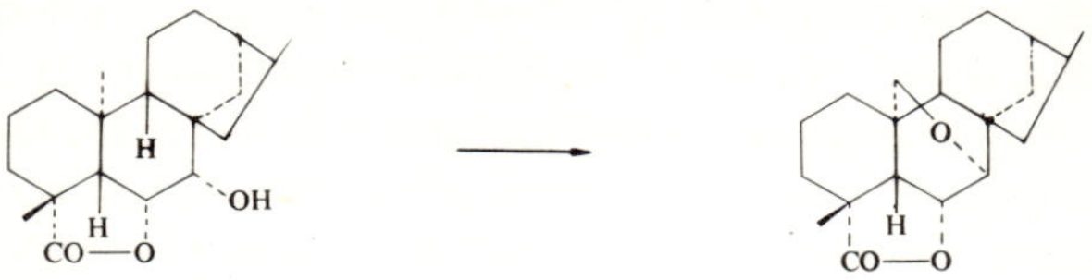

XLV XLVI

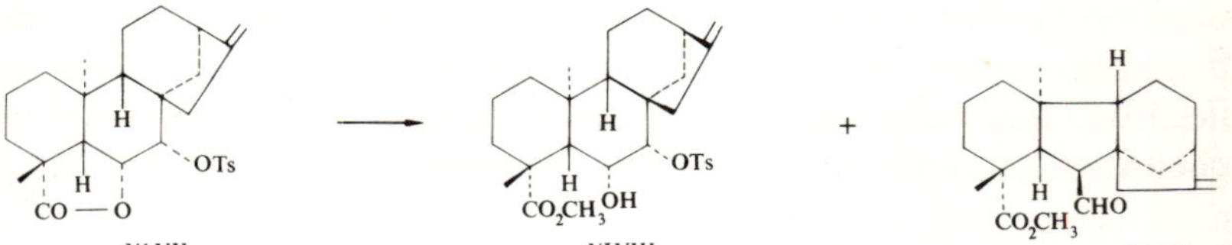

XLVII XLVIII XLIX

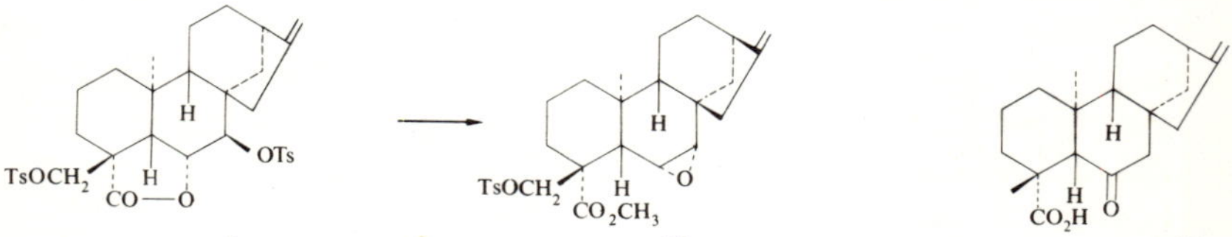

L LI LII

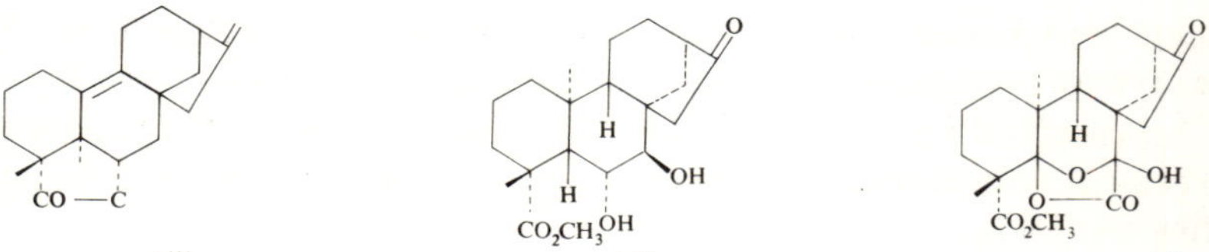

LIII LIV LV

6-ketones (e.g. LII). Alternatively, treatment with phosphorus pentachloride gave a mixture of the 6-keto-acid (LII) and enol-lactone (XLII) together with a γ-lactone assigned the structure (LIII). Typically of a hindered ketone, reduction of the 6-ketone with sodium borohydride led to the axial alcohol. Relactonization of the 6-hydroxy-acid provided[68] a synthesis of kaurenolide.

Acetylation of both $6\alpha,7\alpha$ and $6\alpha,7\beta$ glycols gave the 7-mono acetates. Similar treatment of a 6α,19-diol gave the 19-mono acetate.[68] Oxidation[69] of the $6\alpha,7\beta$ glycol (LIV) led to a diosphenol (XL), a dicarboxylic acid (XLI) and a lactonol (LV). The latter as a β-keto ester readily decarboxylated with alkali.

2.5. *Some Aspects of the Chemistry of Ring D of (−)-Kaurene and the Kaurenolides*

Oxidation of ring D of (−)-kaurene and the kaurenolides[69,70] takes place from the α-face of the molecule. Thus both kaurene and isokaurene form 16α,17 and the $15\alpha,16\alpha$-epoxides respectively. Although reduction of both epoxides with lithium aluminium hydride gave kauran-16α-ol, the 15,16-epoxide also gave kaur-16-en-15α-ol.[46] In contrast to the phyllocladene series rearrangement of the 15,16-epoxide with magnesium bromide led to the allylic alcohol, kaur-16-en-15α-ol rather than 15-ketone. In the case of phyllocladene the conversion of C-15 to a trigonal centre involves the release of the steric compression of the angular methyl group. Attack from the less hindered face of the molecule is reflected in the action of methyl magnesium iodide on (—)-17-norkauran-16-one which leads to the 16-epimer of kauranol (kauran-16β-ol). Similarly hydroboronation of (—)-kaurene gave the kauran-17-ol, whilst osmylation led to the 16α,17-diols. In the case of the kaurenolides this was accompanied by some oxidation at position 7. Oxidation of both (—)-kaurene and 7-hydroxykaurenolide with potassium permanganate gave the 16α,17-glycol, 16α-hydroxy 17-acids and the norketone.

Since ozonolysis of the terminal methylene was accompanied by the formation of δ-lactones, the two-step procedure through the glycol and periodate cleavage formed a more satisfactory route to the norketone. In the case of both kaurene and 7-hydroxykaurenolide a 17-seco carboxylic acid (e.g. LVI) was also isolated from the ozonolysis reaction. The δ-lactone (LVII) underwent isomerization to a γ-lactone (LVIII).

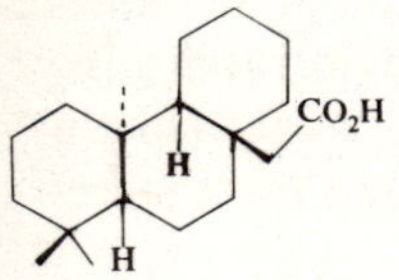

LVI 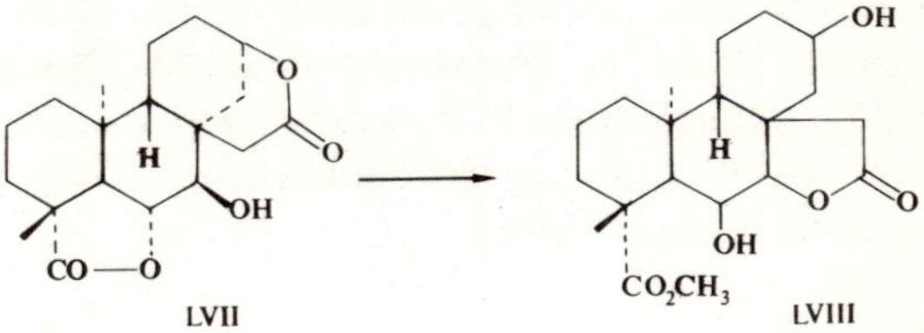 LVII LVIII

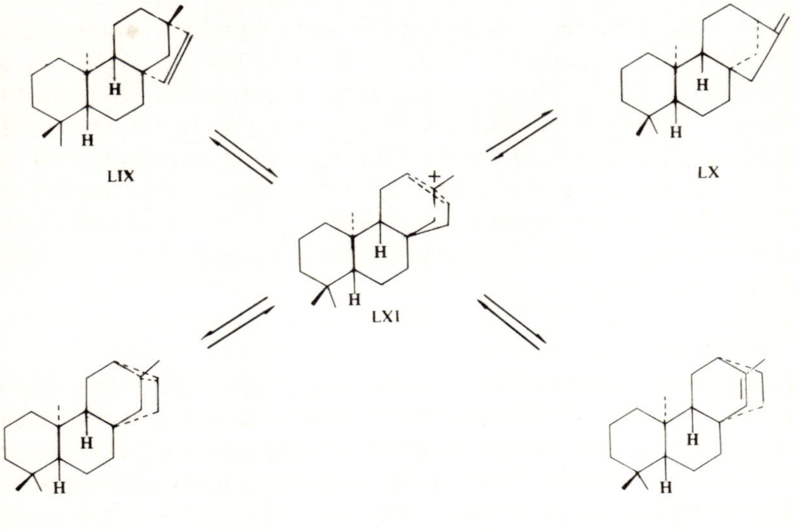

LIX LX

LXI

LXII LXIII

Bromination of isokaurene with *N*-bromosuccinimide led to allylic attack with the formation of 17-bromokaur-15-ene as the major product and curiously a small amount of 13-bromokaur-15-ene.[29] Like isophyllocladene, isokaurene was hydroxylated on the allylic methyl group during the Prévost reaction.[48] Photo-sensitized autoxidation of kaurene[71] gave kaur-15-en-17-ol and the corresponding carboxylic acid whilst isokaurene gave kaur-16-en-15α-ol.

Considerable interest has been attached to the formation of the carbonium ion (LXI) implicit[72] in the biosynthesis of the various tetracyclic skeleta. Thus the acid-catalysed isomerization of stachene (LIX) with hydrogen chloride in acetonitrile led[73] to a mixture of kaurene (LX) and iso-kaurene. This study has been facilitated by the gas chromatography of these hydrocarbons. Similarly rearrangement of stachene epoxide[74] and its relatives with boron trifluoride etherate leads to compounds of the kaurene series. Solvolysis of the 16-exo-toluene-*p*-sulphonate derived from beyerol also leads[75] to the formation of the kaurene skeleton. The acid-catalysed isomerization[76] of (—)-trachylobane (LXII) again produced compounds of the stachene, (—)-isoatisirene (LXIII) and kaurene series. The generation of a similar carbonium ion arises during several other reactions, for example, the steviol-isosteviol and garryfoline-cuauchichicine rearrangements. The latter has been shown[71] by model studies in the kaurene series to be accompanied by a stereospecific hydride shift.

2.6. *Kauranol*

The tertiary alcohol kauran-16α-ol (γ-kaurene, γ-podocarprene[6] or β-cryptomerene)[55] was isolated from an aged sample of kaurene hydrochloride[11] and subsequently from *Gibberella fujikuroi.*[53] It has also been found in *Trachylobium verrucosum.*[77] The hydroxly group has been assigned[44,46] the 16α-configuration on the basis of its formation on reduction of the 16α,17-epoxide and the 17-monotoluene-*p*-sulphonate of kaur-16α,17-diol. Its epimer has been prepared by the action of methyl magnesium iodide on (—)-17-norkauran-16-one.[70] The methyl and ethyl ethers have been isolated from the action of methanolic and ethanolic sulphuric acid on (—)-kaurene.[71]

2.7. *The Kaurene Acids*

The resin of *Ricinocarpus stylosus*, a member of the *Euphorbiaceae* contains a number of kaurane derivatives[78] the simplest of which is (—)-kaur-16-en-19-oic acid (LXIV). This acid has also been isolated[79] from *Gibberella fujikuroi.* Its structure was revealed by interrelationship with (—)-16β-kauran-19-oic acid, obtained from 7-hydroxykaurenolide. (—)-Kaur-16-en-19-oic acid was partially synthesized from 7-hydroxykaurenolide.[80] Oxidation of the kaurenolide gave a ketone which underwent hydrogenolysis with calcium in liquid ammonia to form 7-oxokaur-16-en-19-oic acid. Wolff–Kishner reduction of the latter gave the required acid (LXIV). This acid, which has been synthesized, showed some gibberellin-like activity with dwarf corn.[81]

The two major components of the resin were 16α-(—)-kauran-17,19-dioic acid (LXV) and the corresponding 19-alcohol (LXVI). They were inter-related by oxidation. The two carboxyl groups of the acid differed in their reactivity. Thus methylation under Fischer Spier conditions gave the 17-methyl ester whilst diazomethane gave a dimethyl ester. This could be saponified to 19-monomethyl ester. Evidence for the kauranoid structure of these acids was obtained by degradation of the ester of (LXVI). This was submitted to the Barbier–Wieland degradation to give a cyclo-pentanone (ν_{max} 1743 cm^{-1}). The diphenylethylene intermediate in this degradation was also oxidized to a 19-aldehyde, and the latter subjected to Wolff–Kishner reduction. Cleavage of the double bond then gave authentic (—)-17-norkauran-16-one. Alternatively the 17,19-diol obtained by reduction of the 17,19-dimethyl ester, was oxidized to a dialdehyde and then subjected to Wolff–Kishner reduction to give β-dihydro-(—)-kaurane. [16α-(—)-kaurane]. The same hydrocarbon was obtained from the 17,19-ditoluene-*p*-sulphonate by substitution to form the dibenzyl thio-ether. Hence the carboxyl group at C(16) is in the more stable (exo)-orientation. By careful attention to the reaction conditions it was possible to effect stepwise substitution at C-17 by the mercaptide ion. Desulphurization with Raney nickel and saponification then gave the 19-alcohol (LXVII) which had previously been obtained from steviol[59] and 7-hydroxykaurenolide.[57] This correlation with steviol and 7-hydroxykaurenolide established the location of the second hindered carboxyl group at C-19. 16α(—)-Kauran-17-oic acid has been prepared[70] from (—)-kaurene by rearrangement of the 16,17-epoxide with magnesium bromide-etherate followed by chromium trioxide oxidation.

A triol isolated from the same plant source was shown to be (—)-16α,17,19-trihydroxykaurane (LXVIII) by oxidation to (—)-16-oxo-17-norkauran-19-oic acid. The 16α configuration of the tertiary hydroxyl group was established by resynthesis from (—)-16-oxo-17-norkauran-19-ol. The ketol was converted to the 16-olefin by the Wittig reaction and the 19-acetate then hydroxylated from the α-face of the molecule with osmium tetraoxide. This gave on saponification a single triol identical to the natural material.

A further dihydroxy-acid isolated from the resin has been assigned[82] the structure of 1α,19-dihydroxy-16α-(—)-kauran-17-oic acid (LXIX). Its kauranoid carbon skeleton was demonstrated by oxidation and subsequent reduction of the 1-ketone to the known dimethyl 16α-(—)-kauran-17,

19-dioate. The position of the secondary hydroxy at C-1 was established by bromination of the C-1 ketone and treatment of the bromo derivative with collidine when a 19-2-γ-lactone was formed. This together with the nuclear magnetic resonance spectrum also served to locate the additional oxygen atom. The stereochemistry was assigned on the basis of the multiplicity of C-1-H resonance. The isolation of compounds with a C-1 hydroxy (cf. songorine) has some significance in view of the biosynthesis of the grayanotoxins.

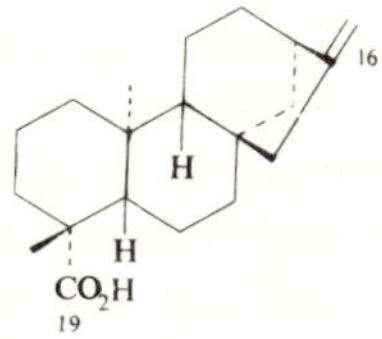

LXIV 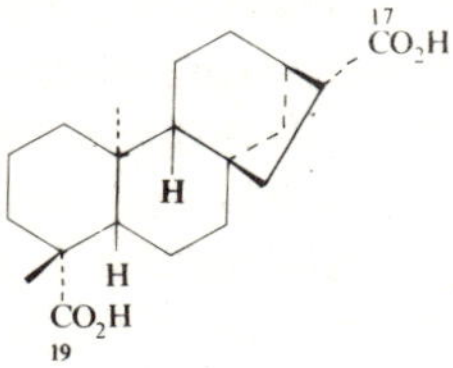 LXV 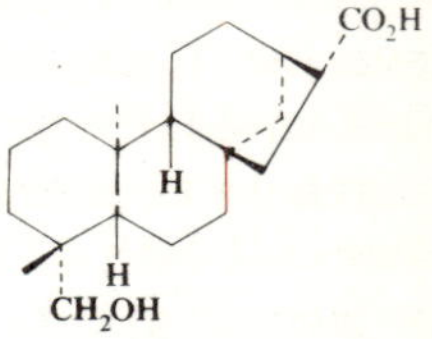 LXVI

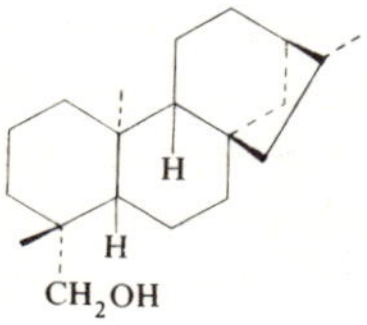

LXVII 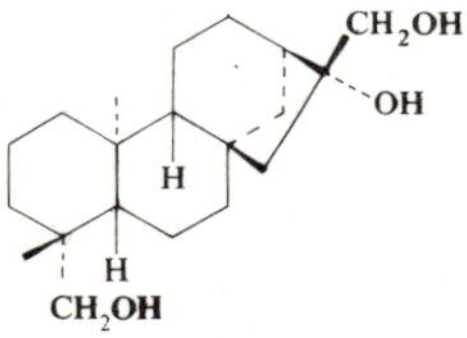 LXVIII 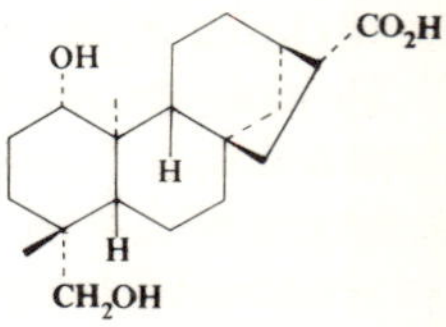 LXIX

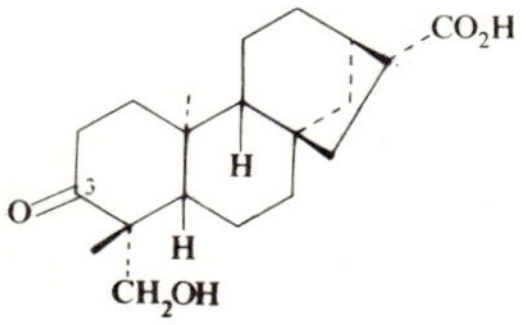

LXX 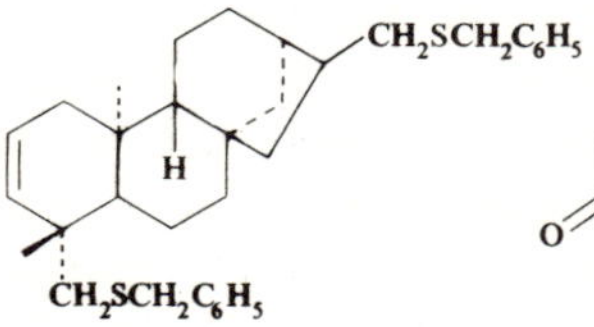 LXXI 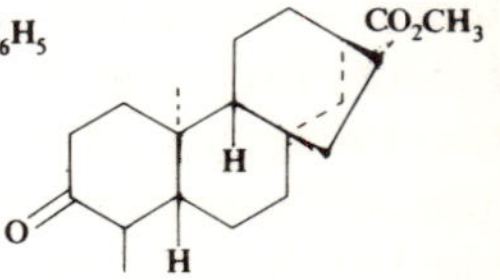 LXXII

The isolation[83] from a related species of *Beyeria brevifolia* of a kauranoid hydroxy-keto-acid (LXX), its acetate, and the corresponding triol has been recorded. The triol was reduced to 16α-(−)-kaurane through its trimethane-sulphonate. The latter when treated with sodium benzyl mercaptide underwent substitution accompanied by elimination to give the unsaturated dibenzyl thio-ether (LXXI). Reduction of the latter gave 16α-(−)-kaurane. The position of the oxygen functions on this skeleton were determined by oxidative studies. Thus the hydroxy-keto-acid was esterified and oxidized to an aldehydo-keto ester which when treated with mild alkali, afforded a norketo-ester (LXXII). Whereas the nuclear magnetic resonance spectrum of the parent keto-aldehyde showed two methyl groups at quaternary positions, the spectrum of the norketone showed a methyl singlet and a doublet thus indicating the presence of an oxygen substituent at C-3 and another on one of the geminal groups. The presence of a 1:3 glycol in the triol was confirmed by the formation of an ethylidene derivative. The location of the third oxygen function at C-17 was demonstrated by the multiplicity of the corresponding aldehyde resonance, revealing the presence of the —CH—CHO grouping. The stereochemistry at C-4 followed from the position of the corresponding aldehyde and acetoxymethyl resonances in the nuclear magnetic resonance spectrum which fell within the range found for axial substituents in similar environments.[84] Furthermore, the acetoxy-keto-ester of (LXX) was converted via its ethylene thio-ketal to the known acetoxy-ester derived from 19-hydroxy-(—)-kauran-17-oic acid (LXVI).

The optical rotatory dispersion curve of the norketone (LXXII) showed a strong negative Cotton effect and was a near mirror image of the curves obtained for 4α-methyl-3-keto 5α-steroids. The occurrence of beyerol with a stachene skeleton in a related *Beyeria* sp. is of considerable interest in the light of the suggestion that these skeleta have a common tricyclic precursor.

Related to these acids is the alcohol, (—)-kaur-16-ene-3α,19-diol which was isolated[85] along with 16α-(—)-kaurane-3α,17,19-triol from a variety of *Beyeria leschenaultii*. The diol has also been isolated from *Helichrysum dendroideum*[140] and, as its 19-succinate, from *Goodenia ramellii.*[141] The 1:3 relationship of the hydroxyl groups in the diol was established by oxidation to the aldehydo-ketone which reacted with both acid or alkali to give a norketone now containing a secondary methyl resonance. The structure of the diol was confirmed by hydroboration of the ethyidene derivative to 16β-hydroxymethyl group. This was oxidized and the methyl ester equilibrated with base to give as the major product, methyl 3α, 19-ethylidene dioxy-16α-(—)-kauran-17-oate which had been previously obtained from the triol. Abbeokutone, isolated from *Didy-mosalpinx abbeokutae*, has been shown[142] to be 3-oxo-(—)-kauran-16,17-diol.

15β-Hydroxy-(—)-kaur-16-en-19-oic acid has been isolated[143] from *Phebalium rude* and, as its acetate, from *Xylopia aethiopica.*[144]

2.8. *Steviol*

The very sweet extract known as Coa-éhé obtained from the Paraguayan plant, *Stevia rebaudiana*, contains the glycoside, stevioside.[86,87] Whilst enzymatic hydrolysis of this gave three moles of glucose[88,89] and the aglycone,[90] steviol $C_{20}H_{30}O_3$ (LXXIII). Acidic hydrolysis gave an isomer, isosteviol (LXXIV). Hydrolysis[89] of the glycoside with base gave steviobioside which was weakly acidic and hence one of the glucose residues was attached to a carboxyl group. The biose residue is a relatively rare 1,2′-disaccharide attached to the 13-hydroxyl. The carbon skeleton of the aglycone was established[90] by dehydrogenation to pimanthrene and by deoxygenation[91] to the 16-epimeric(—)-kauranes. The 16-epimeric dihydro derivatives of steviol were separated. The methyl esters were reduced to diols and then oxidized to the 19-aldehydes which were in turn reduced to the methyl group. The bridgehead hydroxyl was removed by replacement with bromine using phosphorus pentabromide and subsequent reduction with Raney nickel to give the hydrocarbon. Stevanes A and B were subsequently[58, 59, 92] shown to be the epimeric 16-kauranes. Ozonolysis of steviol gave formaldehyde and a

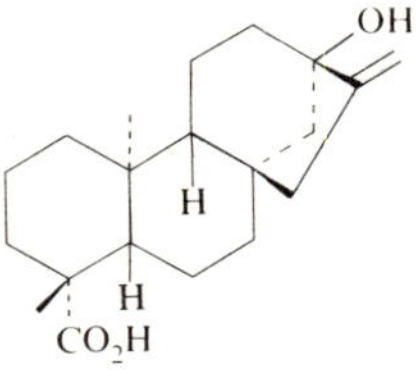

LXXIII

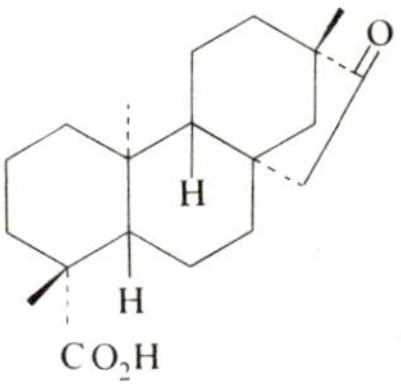

LXXIV

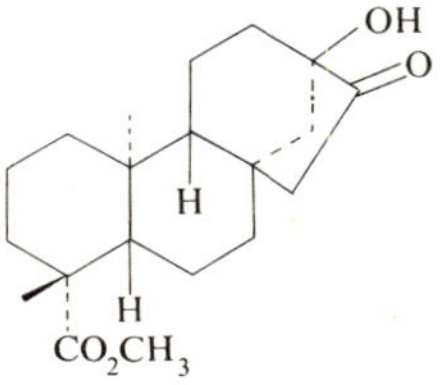

LXXV

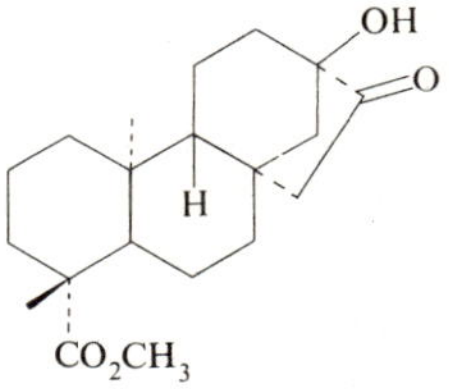

LXXVI

mixture of a ketol (LXXV) and the corresponding keto-acid. This established the position of the hydroxyl group. The steviol–isosteviol rearrangement which is analogous to the allogibberic acid rearrangement (see Chapter 3) is a Wagner–Meerwein rearrangement involving the inversion of ring D. The interrelationship of garryfoline with α-dihydro-(—)-kaurene and the anodic decarboxylation of isostevic acid[93] eliminated the possibility of an angular 10-carboxyl group whilst the pK^*_{MCS} of a number of derivatives placed the carboxyl group as an axial substituent at position 4.

The ketol from steviol showed[59] an optical rotatory dispersion curve with a Cotton effect comparable with that of (—)-17-norkauran-16-one and hence ring D was assigned a β-configuration. Treatment of the ketol (LXXV) with sodium methoxide or butyl lithium brought about rearrangement to the more stable trans-*anti*-trans backbone. This isoketol (LXXVI) showed a negative Cotton effect. Both these ketols were cleaved with solium periodate to keto-acids. The sign and amplitude of their Cotton effects allowed the assignment of the 9β-H configuration to steviol. In view of the relationship to (–)-kaurane this provided one major piece of evidence for the stereochemistry of the latter. The photolysis of N-iodoamides derived from kauran-19-oic acid led to 19-20-δ-lactones.[145] The 20-methyl group may also be functionalized from C-6.

2.9. *(–)-Kaur-16-en-18-oic Acid*

(–)-Kaur-16-en-18-oic acid and 3α-acetoxy-(–)-kaur-16-en-18-oic acid were isolated[77,94] along with the pentacyclic trachylobane diterpenoids from "Zanzibar Copal" a resin isolated from *Trachylobium verrucosum*. The carbon skeleton of these acids was established by reduction to (–)-kaurene. The nuclear magnetic resonance spectrum of the corresponding 18-alcohol showed resonances appropriate to an equatorial group.[84] Further evidence for the stereochemistry of ring D was obtained by ozonolysis to give a norketone with a positive Cotton effect. Cleavage of ring D through the δ-lactone, hydrolysis to the hydroxy-ester followed by oxidation gave a keto-ester with a positive Cotton effect. The structure of 3α-acetoxy-(–)-kaur-16-en-18-oic acid was based on its relationship with the pentacyclic diterpene, acetoxy-trachylobanic acid.

2.10. *Cafestol and Kahweol*

Cafestol (LXXVII) forms one of the main constituents[95,96] of the unsaponifiable part of coffee bean oil, and is accompanied by small amounts of related triene, kahweol (LXXVIII). Some of the earlier work is confused through contamination of cafestol with this triene which is removed by reduction with sodium in alcohol. Initial studies were prompted by the erroneous report[96] of oestrogenic activity and a possible relationship to the steroids. Thus cafestol was shown[97,98] to contain two double bonds by perphthalic acid titration and hydrogenation whilst the oxygen atoms were accounted for in an α-glycol and an oxide ring. The Swiss group of workers,[99] who subsequently suggested[100] a relationship to the diterpenes, showed that it contained a tertiary:primary α-glycol, accounting for two of the three oxygen atoms. Thus dehydration with zinc oxide gave an aldehyde whilst oxidation with lead tetraacetate gave formaldehyde and a norketone, epoxy-norcafestadienone (LXXIX).

The attachment of this glycol to a five-numbered ring was established by oxidation of the norketone with sodium hypiodite to form a dicarboxylic acid which on treatment with acetic anhydride gave an anhydride rather than a ketone. Hence by application of Blanc's rule this ring was five membered—a feature confirmed[101] by the infrared spectrum of the norketone. One of the carboxyl groups of this acid was relatively hindered[102] and hence attached to a tertiary centre.

The combination of the inert third oxygen atom and the two double bonds on a furan ring was established on a number of pieces of evidence.

Thus exhaustive hydrogenation led[100] to a mixture of products including two epimeric tetrahydrofurans, and arising by hydrogenolysis, two epimeric secondary alcohols and a primary alcohol. Cleavage of the ring D glycol and oxidation of the two alcohols gave a dione which on Wolff–Kishner reduction gave a hydrocarbon, norcafestane—a degradation carried out in the unfulfilled expectation of a link with the steroids. Chromium trioxide oxidation of the tetrahydrofuran afforded a lactone in turn hydrolysed and oxidized to a lactonol (LXXX). Thus the tetrahydrofuran contained a primary: secondary oxide ring. Alternatively the furan formed[103] both a mono- and diepoxide with monoperphthalic acid. Hydrogenation of the latter gave a lactonol related to the oxidation product described above. Hydrolysis of mono epoxide and acetylation led to an enol-acetate (LXXXI).

The relationship of the furan ring to the rest of the molecule came from several pieces of evidence. Cafestol readily formed a maleic anhydride adduct[104–107] which was cleaved with acid and oxidized[104] to mellophanic acid (benzene-1:2:3:4-tetracarboxylic acid). The furan ring was thus

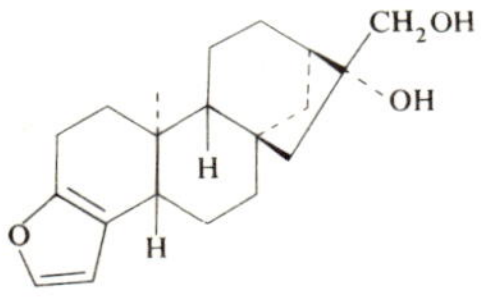

LXXVII 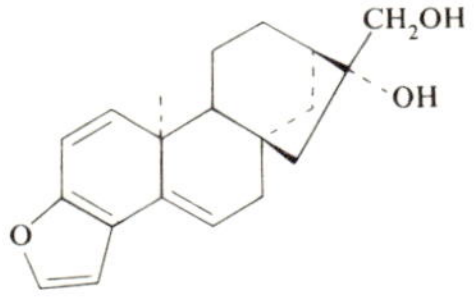 LXXVIII 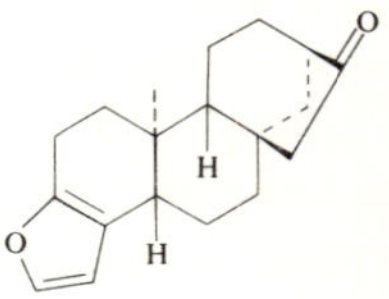 LXXIX

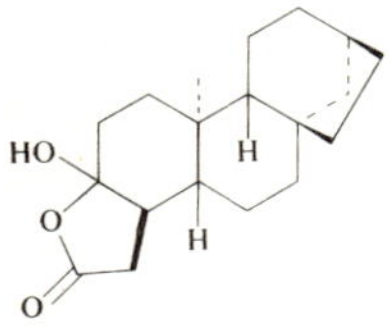

LXXX 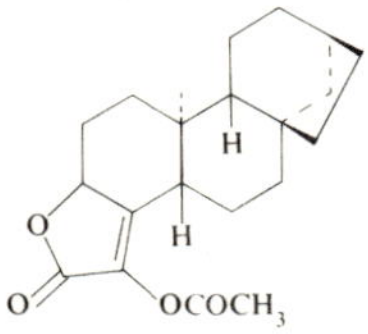 LXXXI 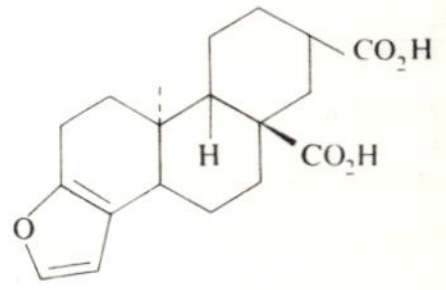 LXXXII

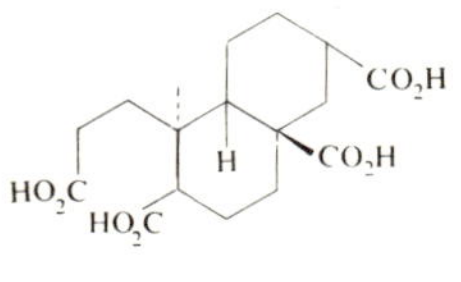

LXXXIII 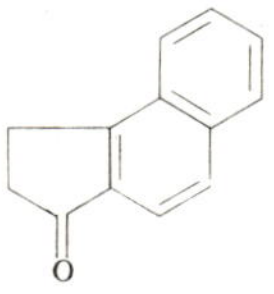 LXXXIV 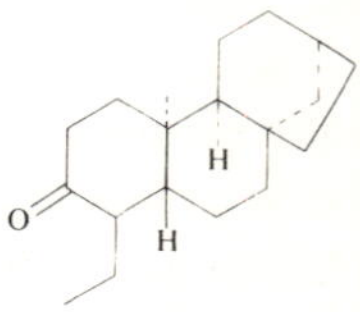 LXXXV

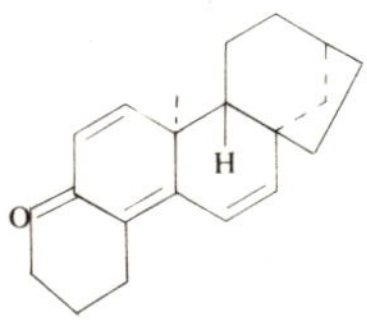

LXXXVI 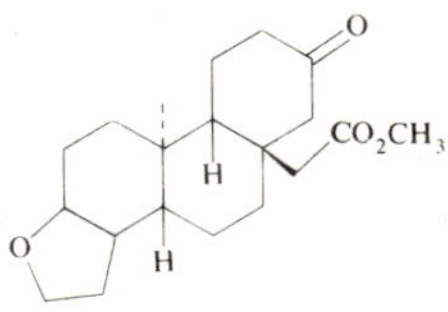 LXXXVII 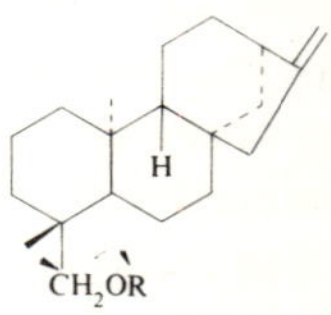 LXXXVIII

2:3 disubstituted. That the substituents were part of a six-membered ring appeared from ozonolysis experiments. Ozonolysis of the furan ring gave[104] a dicarboxylic acid which on treatment with acetic anhydride gave a ketone. The same ketone was obtained by treatment of the dimethyl ester with sodium. It formed a monobenzylidene derivative whilst infrared evidence showed[101] it to be a cyclopentanone.

The position of the furan ring on the perhydrophenanthrene backbone was established by cleavage of ring D of epoxynorcafestadienone (LXXIX) to dicarboxylic acid (LXXXII) and dehydrogenation of this to form 1-ethylphenanthra-2-ol.[108, 111]

Ozonolysis of the furan ring in epoxynorcafestadienone, followed by pyrolysis[109] of the resultant dicarboxylic acid produced a second cyclopentanone with an additional α-methylene group. Dehydrogenation of this produced a benzindanone whilst dehydrogenation of the corresponding seco ring D tetracarboxylic acid (LXXXIII) gave 1-ethyl-2-methylnaphthalene[110] and the benzindanone (LXXXIV). At one time this was also quoted as support for an angular methyl group at position 5. However, many examples are now known of alkyl group migration during dehydrogenation experiments and this aspect of cafestol chemistry is no longer a subject of dispute. Thus cafestol contained a 1,2-furanoperhydrophenanthrene backbone. Since the infrared spectrum of the C_{19} epoxynorcafestadienone showed[108, 111] the presence of only one C-methyl group, the five-menbered ring must share three nuclear carbon atoms, i.e. it must be attached 1:3 to the perhydrophenanthrene nucleus. Furthermore, in experiments aimed at elucidating the size of ring D, it was noted that the carboxyl groups of the dicarboxylic acid differed greatly in their reactivity consistent with the location of one at a ring junction. Deuteration experiments and the resistance of bromoepoxynorcafestanone to dehydrobromination suggested an attachment of ring D as in phyllocladene.

Hydrogenolysis of the furan ring in epoxynorcafestadiene and subsequent oxidation of the alcohol produced a ring A ketone (LXXXV). The reduction of this ketone with both lithium aluminium hydride and lithium in liquid ammonia gave[42] equatorial products comparable with 4-ethylcholestan-3-one rather than friedelin whilst on bromination and dehydrobromination a trienone (LXXXVI) was produced. This supported placing the angular methyl group at position 10 rather than 5 and also limited the position of ring D. The similarity of the positive Cotton effect in the optical rotatory dispersion curve of the norketone, epoxynorcafestanone, to that of (+)-17-norphyllocladan-16-one apart from supporting its structure, permitted the assignment of a β-ring D to cafestol. The negative sign of the Cotton effect in the O.R.D. curve of the 3-ketone (LXXXV) implied an antipodal A/B fusion.

The stereochemistry of the B/C/D fusion was studied[113] by Baeyer–Villiger oxidation of the norketone to a δ-lactone and oxidation of this to a keto-ester (LXXXVII) which showed a positive Cotton effect comparable with that of a similar compound derived from phyllocladene. Hence the unique trans-*syn*-trans backbone with a boat ring B was initially assigned to cafestol. However, the generalization that there is a *trans* relationship between the angular methyl group and 9-hydrogen led to a re-examination[114] of the problem. X-ray analysis of α-bromo-epoxynorcafestanone revealed that the 9-hydrogen atom is β. Finally, the stereochemistry at C-16 was defined[115] by resynthesis of the glycol involving a Wittig reaction on epoxynorcafestanone, and osmylation of the resultant olefin. Hence the structure and stereochemistry (LXXVII) was assigned to cafestol. The generation of the furan ring can be visualized by assuming a Wagner–Meerwein rearrangement (LXXXVIII) parallel to that found in the formation of methylabietin from abietinol.[116]

On the basis of the ultraviolet spectrum and its reduction [101,102] to cafestol, kahweol has been assigned[112,117] the structure (LXXVIII).

Corymbol, a triol from *Turbina corymbosa* has been shown[118] to possess a similar α-glycol system and is formulated as (—)-6β, 16α, 17-trihydroxy-kaurane. It is related to turbincorytin isolated from the same plant.

2.11. *Atractyligenin*

Atractyligenin, the aglycone of atractyloside,[119] from *Atractylis gummifiera*, has been shown to be a norditerpene probably[119] possessing the kauranoid structure (LXXXIX). The oxygen functions were accounted

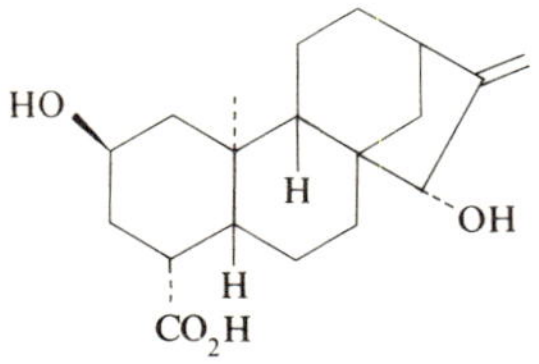

HO H OH H CO_2H

LXXXIX

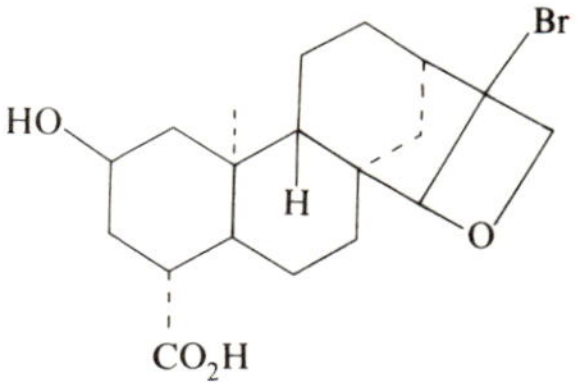

Br HO H O CO_2H

XC

for in carboxyl and two secondary hydroxyl groups. Dehydrogenation experiments gave a number of phenanthrenes including retene, indicating a diterpenoid carbon skeleton. The nuclear magnetic resonance spectrum indicated the presence of a single tertiary methyl group (τ9·08) and suggested that one of the hydroxyl groups (CH—OH at τ 6·14) was allylic to the terminal methylene (τ 4·92 and 4·76). In the corresponding dihydro compound this CH·OH resonance appears as a doublet at higher field (τ6·75; J = 3·5). In confirmation of this oxidation gave an $\alpha\beta$-unsaturated ketone. Double irradiation experiments demonstrated the position of the other hydroxyl group. Examination of the spectrum showed that the

CH·OH proton (at τ 5·77) appeared as a triplet of triplets—a situation accommodated by equatorial hydroxylation at C-2. The position of the C-4 proton resonance indicated that the carboxyl substituent at that centre was axial in atractyligenin. Furthermore, this centre was epimerized with base. On bromination atractyligenin formed an unusual ether (XC). The C-17 norketone produced by ozonolysis showed a positive Cotton effect typical of a β-oriented ring D. The overall kauranoid stereochemistry has been confirmed by interrelationship with the 16-epimeric-19-nor-(—)-kauranes[146] and with 19-nor-(—)-kauran-18-oic acid.[147]

2.12. *The seco-Ring B Group of Tetracyclic Diterpenes*

A small group of tricyclic diterpenes are known in which ring B of the tetracyclic diterpenes has been cleaved. Their chemistry and substitution differs markedly from that of the other tricyclic diterpenes and

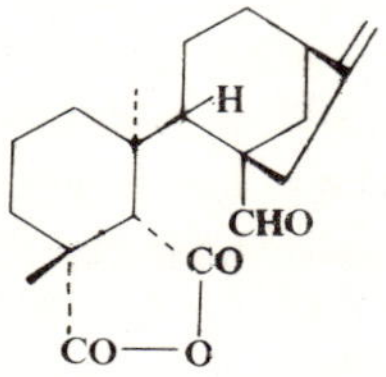

XCI

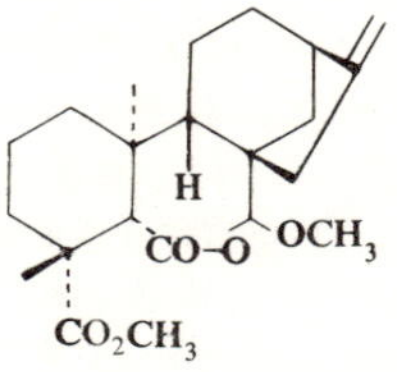

XCII

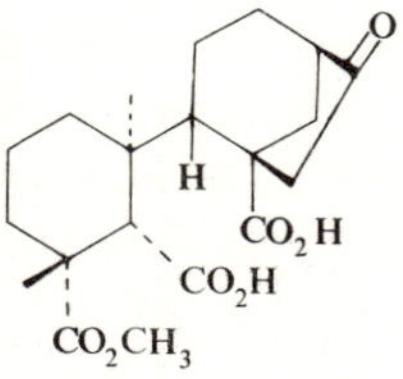

XCIII

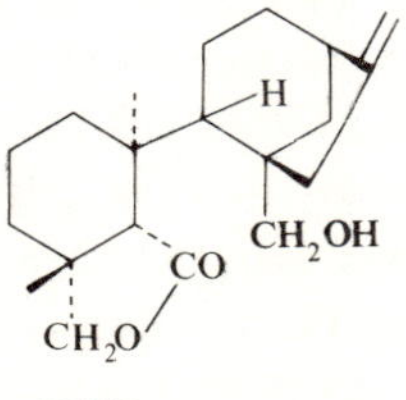

XCIV

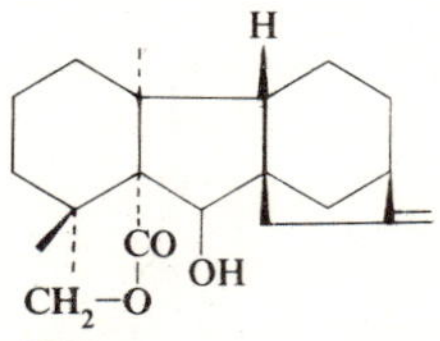

XCV

resembles the tetracyclic diterpenes from which they appear to be biogenetically derived.

Fujenal and fujenoic acid. Fujenal (XCI) occurs[53] along with the kaurenolides, to which it is related, as a diterpenoid metabolite of *Gibberella fujikuroi.* The oxygen functions were characterized by their spectral properties as the relatively rare glutaric anhydride and aldehyde groups.

Oxidation of the latter gave fujenoic acid which was also isolated from the mould. Ozonolysis of the double bond showed[120] that it was attached as a terminal methylene group to a cyclopentane ring.

Treatment of fujenal with methanolic hydrogen chloride or with methanol in a sealed tube at 160° gave a group of pseudo-esters (e.g. XCII) thus relating the anhydride and aldehyde functions. Mild acid hydrolysis of the 17-nor-16-ketone of the pseudo-ester (XCII) served to distinguish between the ester and methoxyketal functions and converted the latter to a lactonol. Oxidation then gave a dicarboxylic acid (XCIII), which was also obtained from 7-hydroxykaurenolide thus defining the structure and stereochemistry of fujenal. Fujenal is reduced by lithium aluminium hydride to the γ-lactone (XCIV) which is then oxidized to the aldehyde. Treatment of this with base led[121] to cyclization and the formation of a compound of the gibbane skeleton (XCV).

2.13. *Enmein*

The complex bitter principle, enmein (isodonin)(XCVI) was isolated[122] in Japan from *Isodon trichocarpus* and shown[123] to contain a δ-lactone, hemiacetal, cisoid $\alpha\beta$-unsaturated ketone and a cyclohexanol as the oxygen functions. Structural studies have culminated in the recent[124] proposal (XCVI) which was substantiated[125] by X-ray analysis of a bromoacetyl derivative. The relationship of the oxygen functions was determined by a series of oxidation and elimination reactions whilst cleavage of the 9–10 bond gave identifiable fragments. In this highly oxygenated molecule nuclear magnetic resonance spectroscopy played an important part in the later structural work. Some indication of the underlying carbon skeleton was obtained by distillation with baryta which gave 1-ethyl-4-(3,3-dimethylcyclohexyl)-benzene (XCVII). Oxidation of an α-dihydroenmein gave a saturated ketonic-γ-lactone. This, on treatment with alkali gave an acidic $\alpha\beta$-unsaturated ketone (XCVIII) which, whilst it retained the γ-lactone, had lost the δ-lactone function. The new carboxyl group, which therefore corresponded to the δ-lactone of enmein, was lost on pyrolysis of the corresponding saturated ketone, indicating the relationship of rings C and D to ring A and the presence of carbonyl group β to the δ-lactone. Further pyrolysis of the $\alpha\beta$-unsaturated ketone (XCVIII) gave three highly informative fragments [(XCIX) to (CI)].

The following evidence contributed to the structure of ring A. The anomeric proton of the hemiacetal appeared as a doublet in the nuclear magnetic resonance spectrum whilst the multiplicity of the terminal protons of the lactone ring indicated that they belonged to a primary alcohol attached to a quaternary centre. Furthermore this angular group was lost as formaldehyde in a retroaldol reaction. Ozonolysis of the $\alpha\beta$-unsaturated ketone (XCVIII) gave a neutral bis-δ-lactone containing

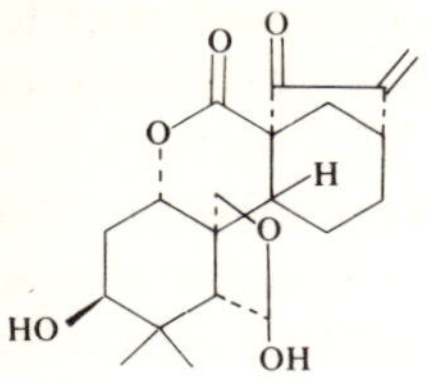

XCVI 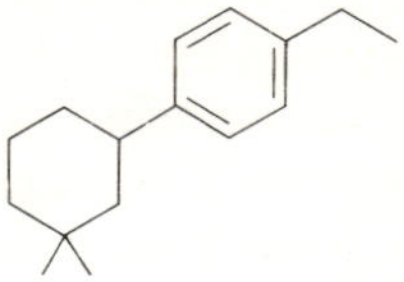 XCVII 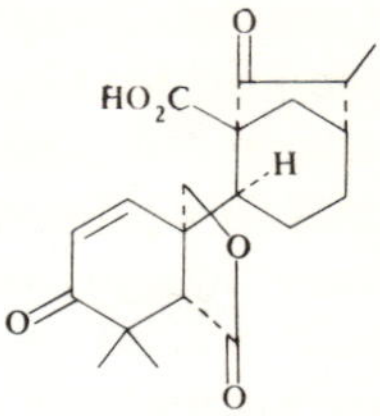 XCVIII

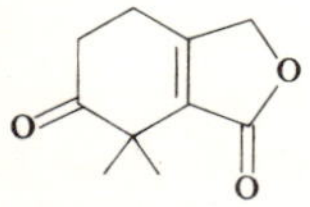

XCIX 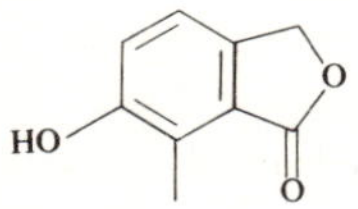 C 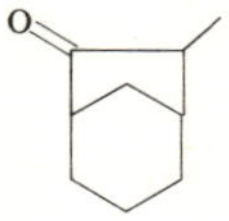 CI

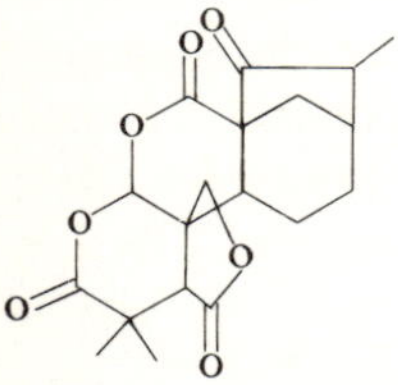

CII 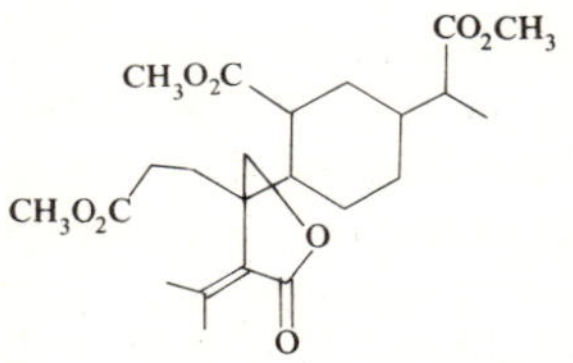 CIII 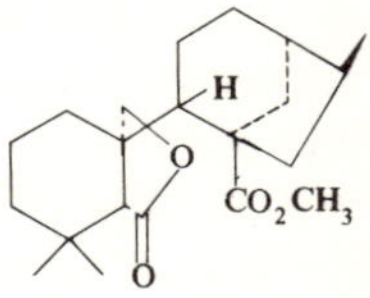 CIV

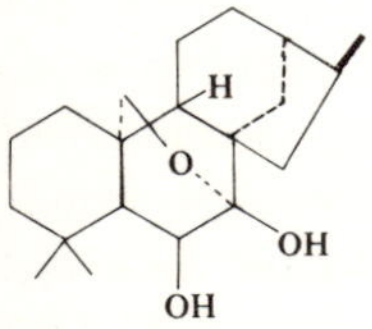

CV 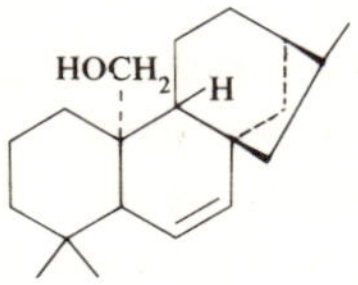 CVI

the fragment (CII). Ring D of the $\alpha\beta$-unsaturated keto-acid (XCVIII) was cleaved under acidic conditions and after hydrogenation, ring A was opened by a Baeyer–Villiger reaction. Both the nuclear magnetic resonance spectrum of the product (CIII) and its ozonolysis to give acetone confirmed the presence of the fragment $(CH_3)_2C{=}C$ and hence a gem-dimethyl group in enmein. On the basis of this and other evidence enmein was therefore assigned the structure (XCVI).

Optical rotatory dispersion measurements indicated that ring D had an α-configuration. The stereochemical consequences of the above degradation further delineated the stereochemistry. The relationship of enmein to the tetracyclic diterpenes can be seen taking compounds of the fujenal type and rotating them about the 9–10 bond. This relationship has been confirmed experimentally.[126, 127] Thus the oxygen functions on rings A and D were removed through their thioketal and mesylates. An acyloin condensation of the ester (CIV) then led to a group of ethers and alcohols comprising mainly (CV). Wolff–Kishner reduction then led to the primary alcohol (CVI) which was in turn reduced to (−)-kaurane. Unsuccessful efforts to transform the lactone (XCIV) derived from fujenal to compounds of the enmein type have shown that the lactone exists primarily as the rotamer (XCIV).[148] Recently a number of compounds related to enmein have been isolated[128] from further *Isodon* sp. Thus trichokaurin and oridonin are kauranoid ring B 6:7-glycols (cf. CV) that are related to possible progenitors of enmein. The enmein series has also been transformed[146] into enantioabietane.

2.14. *The Grayanotoxins*

The toxicity of the leaves of many species of *Rhododendron* and *Kalmia* (e.g. *K. latifolia*, the mountain laurel) and other members of the *Ericaceae* has been described in agricultural records for many years.[129] Grayanotoxin-1 (andromedotoxin or acetyl-andromedol[130]) isolated[131] from *Leucothoe grayana*, is one of the most widespread[132] of these toxic agents. It has also been described[133] as a potent hypotensive agent. The grayanotoxins known at present are related as follows:

$$C_{22}H_{36}O_7 \rightarrow C_{20}H_{34}O_6 + CH_3CO_2H \rightarrow C_{20}H_{32}O_5 + H_2O$$

G. I (CVII, R=Ac) G. III (CVII, R=H) G. II (CVIII)

Although these extracts have been studied for many years, it was not until 1961 that their structures were known with any certainty when two independent degradations were published[134,135] almost simultaneously. Both made use of a similar approach involving the cleavage of ring B. Thus grayanotoxin G. II was shown to possess one double bond, present as a terminal methylene group, together with five hydroxyl

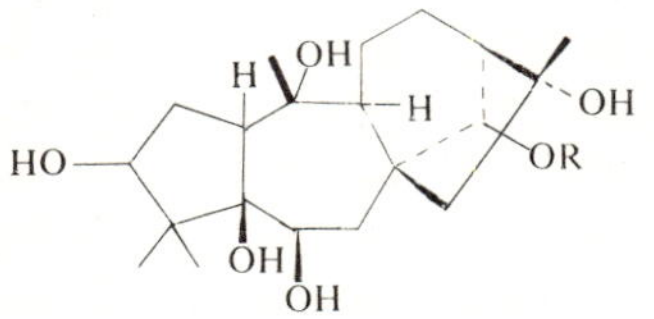

CVII

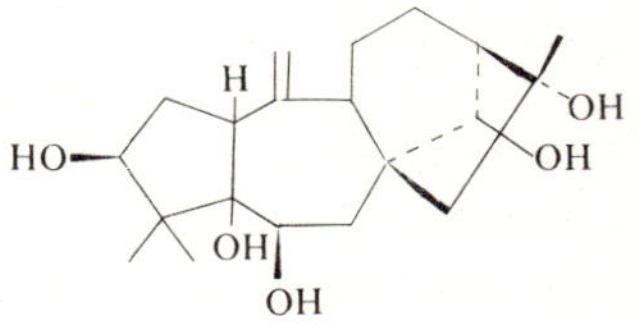

CVIII

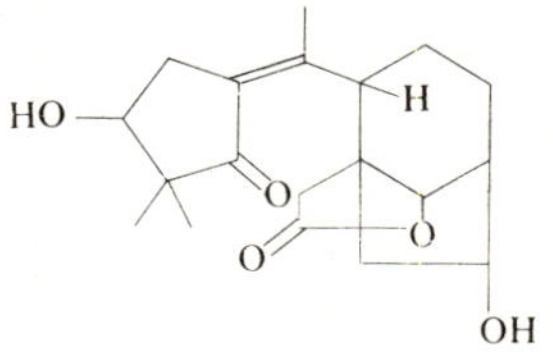

CIX

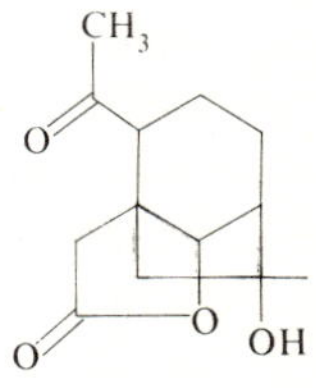

CX

groups, two of which as an α-glycol, readily formed an isopropylidene derivative. Hence grayanotoxin G. II was a tetracyclic penta-ol. Oxidation established that two of the other hydroxyl groups were attached to five-membered rings and that one of these bore an acetyl group in G. I. Treatment of G.II with anhydrous copper sulphate in acetone gave monoisopropylidene anhydro-G. II which, after hydrogenation, was oxidized to a diketone showing the infrared absorption characteristic of cyclopentanones. Alternatively hydrogenation of monoisopropylidene anhydro G. I, and oxidation then gave a monoketone which on Wolff–Kishner reduction and hydrolysis gave an alcohol in which the hydroxyl group was derived from the acetoxyl of G. I. Oxidation then gave a cyclopentanone. Therefore G. II contained a cis α-glycol, one tertiary hydroxyl group which was readily eliminated, and two secondary cyclopentanol hydroxyl groups, one of which was masked as an acetoxyl in G. I. The α-glycol was shown to be secondary:tertiary by fission with lead tetra-acetate or sodium periodate to give a keto-aldehyde.

Both degradations employed the cleavage of ring B. Thus fission of the α-glycol led to the unsaturated keto-γ-lactone (CIX) which on ozonolysis gave two fragments, $\alpha\alpha$-dimethyl-β-acetoxyglutaric acid from ring A and the keto-lactone (CX) from rings C and D. The latter was degraded to 2,5-dicarboxyphenylacetic acid thus marking the points of attachment of rings B and D to ring C. The second degradation made use[136] of a similar approach employing grayanotoxins G. I and G. III. The ring A hydroxyl was linked to the ring B glycol by oxidation to form a cyclopentene-3,5-dione.

The stereochemistry of the grayanotoxins was assigned[137,138] on the basis of evidence in which transannular ether formation reactions played an important part. The optical rotatory dispersion curve of the 16-ketone (CXI) showed a positive Cotton effect, whilst the 14-ketone (CXII) showed a negative Cotton effect. Consequently ring D was assigned a β-configuration. The latter ketone was prepared from isopropylidene G. I by catalytic hydrogenation of the double bonds, removal of the C_3-OH by selective oxidation and Wolff–Kishner reduction followed by further chromic oxide oxidation. Since oxidative cleavage of the $C_{5,6}$ α-glycol leads to ready hemiacetal and lactone formation (CIX) between C_7 and C_{14}, the C_{14}-OR and $C_{7\text{-}8}$ bond must possess a *cis*-relationship with respect to ring D. Confirmation of this C_{14} stereochemistry came from the formation of a diethylidene derivative (CXIII) from G. III involving not only the $C_{5,6}$ α-glycol but also the 1:3 glycol of ring D. Evidence for the stereochemistry at position 9 came from the enolization of the $\alpha\beta$-unsaturated ketone (CIX) to a more stable isomer (i.e. to an isomer in which ring A is an equatorial substituent on ring C). Hence the hydrogen atom at C-9 was assigned a β-configuration in the normal series and the B/C ring junction of the grayanotoxins is *cis* fused characteristic of a kauranoid system. This relationship and the configuration of the C_{10}-OH was also settled[139] by an interesting rearrangement reminiscent of the anthra-steroid rearrangement. Treatment of

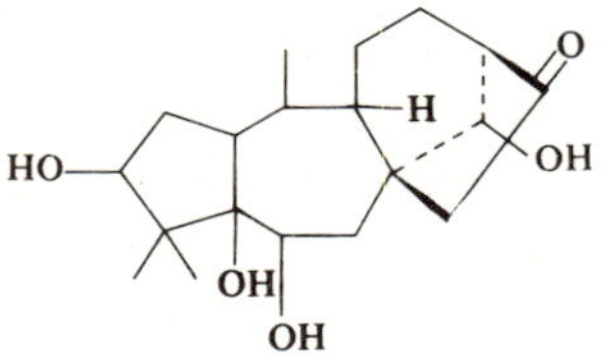

CXI 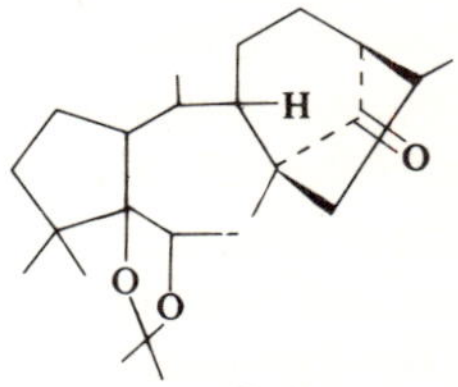 CXII

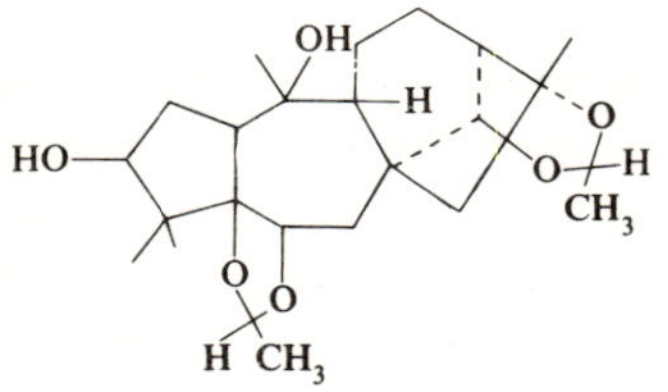

CXIII 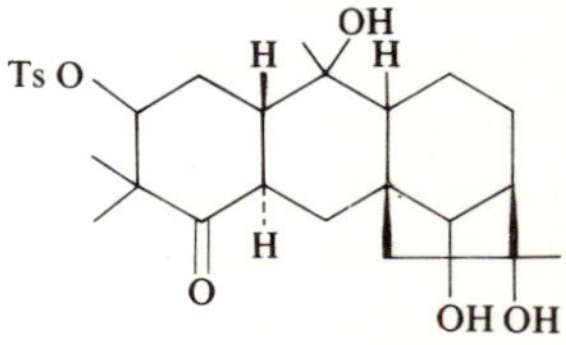 CXIV

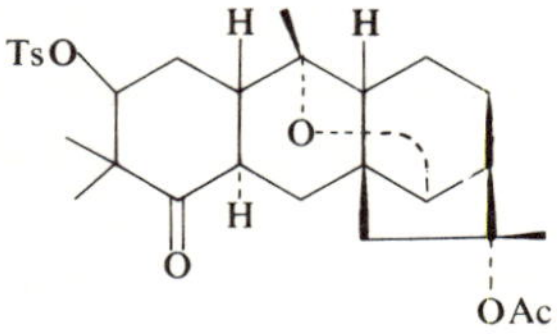

CXV 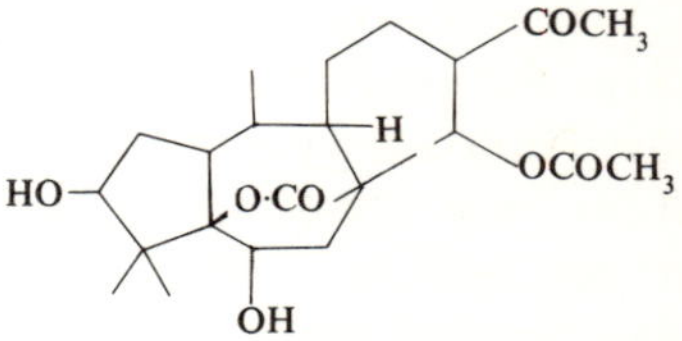 CXVI

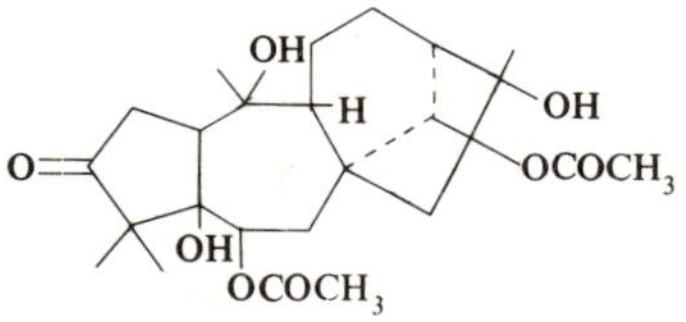

CXVII

G. I with toluene-*p*-sulphonyl chloride in pyridine for 2–3 weeks, gave a mixture of the triol (CXIV) and transannular ether (CXV). The infrared spectra of the products indicated the formation of a cyclohexanone (ν_{max} 1700 and 1710 cm^{-1}) and thus the five–seven membered A/B system had undergone rearrangement to a six–six system. This was attributed to a pinacol rearrangement of the α-glycol in view of the recovery of 6,14-diacetyl G. III under these conditions. The nuclear magnetic resonance spectrum of the ether was compatible with the structure (CXV) particularly in showing five singlet C-methyl resonances (τ8·90, 8·83, 8·70, 8·63, and 7·85) and in the multiplicity of the C_{14}-H resonance at τ5·57. This rearrangement which required an acyl migration from C_{14} to C_{10} provided a very elegant demonstration of the stereochemistry at the asymmetric centres of C_{10} and rings C and D.

Ozonolysis of the $\Delta^{15,16}$ double bond led to the formation of a hemiacetal (CXX) involving the C-5 hydroxyl which was therefore also a β-substituent. Confirmation of this and the assignment of the *cis* A/B fusion came from the optical rotatory dispersion curves of a 3-keto derivative (CXVII) which exhibited a weak negative Cotton effect in contrast to the strong Cotton effects shown by A-nor triterpenes with a *trans* fused system. Consequently the ring fusion was *cis* and the C_1-H was assigned a β-configuration. The stereochemistry of the C_3- and C_6-hydroxyls were assigned making use of Horeau's asymmetric synthesis of α-phenyl butyric acids. The configuration of both hydroxyls was deduced as β. The hydroxyl groups curiously differ in their reactivity. Thus C_6 is acetylated and tosylated prior to C_3 whilst the reverse was true of benzoylation.

The biosynthesis of the grayanotoxins can be envisaged through elimination of a 1-equatorial substituent of a kaurane ring system.

2.15. *The cyclo Kaurane Diterpenes*

The resin of *Trachylobium verrucosum* known as "Madagascan" or "Zanzibar Copal" contains[77] a number of diterpenes. These fall into three classes. Zanzibaric acid possessing a bicyclic labdane skeleton, some kauranoid derivatives (see Section 2.9) and a group of compounds possessing the pentacyclic trachylobane skeleton (CXX). This pentacyclic skeleton represents an interesting stabilized form of the non-classical carbonium ion proposed[72] by Wenkert as an intermediate in the biosynthesis of the tetracyclic diterpenes.

Trachylobanic acid (CXVIII, R = H), the corresponding 3-hydroxy and 3-acetoxy-acid were inter-related by acetylation and by reductive removal of the 3-oxygen function. The latter involved the reduction of the 3-tosylhydrazone with lithium aluminium hydride and furnished an alcohol, trachylobanol which was also isolated from the resin. Oxidation of the 3-hydroxyl to a 3-ketone led to ready decarboxylation indicating a β-hydroxy-acid. The absence of spectral evidence for a double bond indicated that the skeleton was pentacyclic. The nuclear magnetic resonance spectrum of the ester (CXVIII, R = Me) contained two high field proton resonances at τ 9·25 and 9·41 indicative of a cyclopropane ring. Dehydrogenation experiments gave rise to four phenanthrene hydrocarbons: pimanthrene, retene, 1-methyl-6-isopropyl phenanthrene, and 1,7-dimethyl-6-ethyl phenanthrene. The formation of each one of these may be accounted for by a simple fragmentation of the trachylobane skeleton. A relationship with the kauranoid skeleton was achieved by treating the ester (CXVIII, R = Me) with perchloric acid in a mixture of acetic acid and acetic anhydride. This led to the acylated kaurene derivative (CXIX) which was in turn ozonized to form a norketone derived directly from methyl kaur-16-en-18-oic acid.

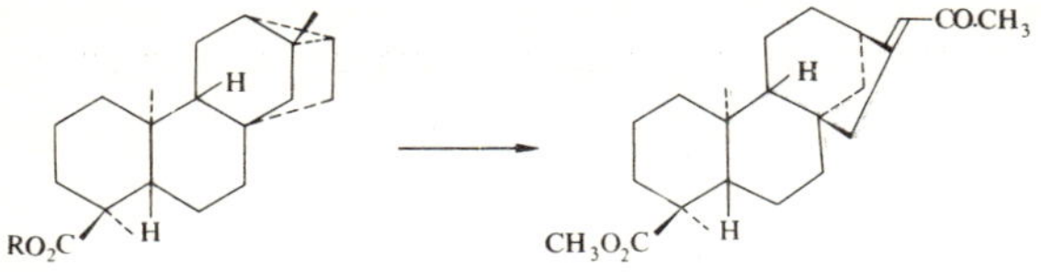

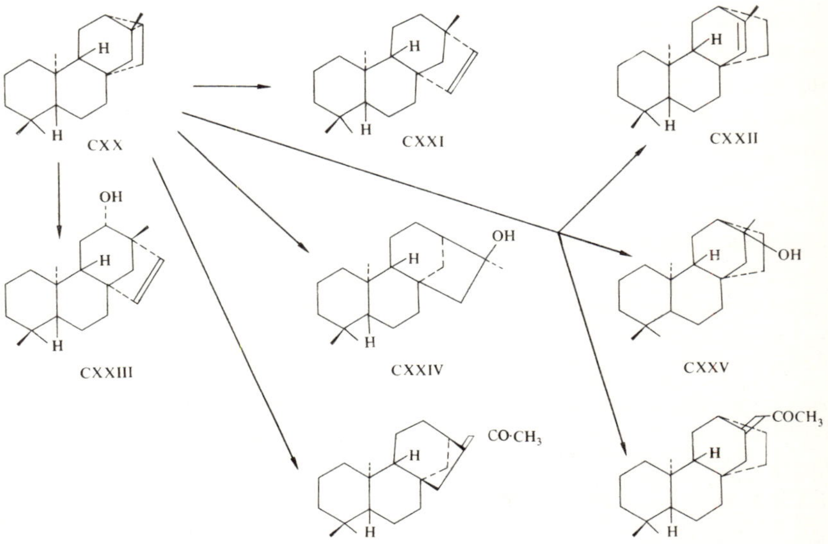

The n.m.r. spectra of the ester-acetate contained a resonance indicative of an axial hydrogen at position 3 and hence an equatorial oxygen function whilst the spectrum of trachylobanol contained resonances at τ 6·86 assigned to an equatorial primary alcohol. The antipodal absolute configuration of the series was obtained by the application of Horeau's method to position 3.

The parent hydrocarbon, trachylobane (CXX), was prepared by oxidation of trachylobanol to the corresponding aldehyde and subsequent Wolff–Kishner reduction. The acid-catalysed cleavage of its cyclopropane ring is of biogenetic interest. Thus (−)-trachylobane on treatment[76] with a mixture of acetic acid and anhydride containing a trace of perchloric acid gave a series of fractions. The hydrocarbon fraction contained stachene (CXXI) and isoatiserene (CXXII). A second fraction contained the acetates of 12α-hydroxy-stachene (CXXIII) and as minor constituents atisan-16-ol (CXXV) and curiously the 16-epimer of kauranol (CXXIV). The third and largest fraction comprised the acylated kaurene and atiserene derivatives (CXXVI) and (CXXVII). Comparable results were obtained through the action of trifluoroacetic acid, and the acetic acid/anhydride–perchloric acid mixture on methyl trachylobanate. During preliminary oxidation studies on 3-acetoxy-methyl trachylobanate an 11-ketone was obtained. This ketone showed a resistance to further reaction comparable with the hindrance shown by 11-position in the steroids.

REFERENCES

1. Sir John Simonsen and D. H. R. Barton, *The Terpenes,* Vol. III, p. 340, Cambridge University Press, London (1951): R. T. Baker and H. G. Smith, *Pines of Australia,* Technological Museum, Sydney, p. 419 (1910).
2. R. T. Aplin, R. C. Cambie and P. S. Rutledge, *Phytochemistry*, **2**, 205 (1963).
3. Cf. H. A. Aitken, *J. Soc. Chem. Ind.*, **48**, 344T (1929).
4. Cf. G. J. Hunter, *J. Soc. Chem. Ind.*, **51**, 394T (1932).
5. L. H. Briggs, *J. N.Z. Inst. Chem.*, **23**, 92 (1959).
6. Cf. K. Nishida and H. Uota, *Bull. Agric. Chem. Soc.* (Japan), **6**, 82 (1930); *J. Agric. Chem. Soc.* (Japan), **6**, 1078 (1930); **7**, 157, 957 (1931) who isolated (—)-kaurene.
7. L. H. Briggs and R. W. Cawley, *J. Chem. Soc.*, 1888 (1948).
8. J. Murray, *J. Appl. Chem.*, **10**, 366 (1960).
9. J. R. Hosking and W. F. Short, *Rec. Trav. Chim.*, **47**, 834 (1928).
10. L. H. Briggs, R. W. Cawley, J. A. Loe and W. I. Taylor, *J. Chem. Soc.*, 956 (1950).
11. J. R. McGimpsey and J. Murray, *J. Appl. Chem.*, **10**, 340 (1960).
12. W. J. Blackie, *J. Soc. Chem. Ind.*, **48**, 357 (1929); **49**, 26 (1930).
13. L. H. Briggs, *J. Chem. Soc.*, 79 (1937).
14. F. H. McDowall and H. J. Finlay, *J. Soc. Chem. Ind.*, **44**, 42 (1925).
15. M. S. Carrie, *J. Soc. Chem. Ind.*, **51**, 367 (1932).
16. B. H. Goudie, *J. Soc. Chem. Ind*., **42**, 357 (1923).
17. H. A. Aitken, *J. Soc. Chem. Ind.*, **47**, 223 (1928).
18. L. H. Briggs and W. I. Taylor, *J. Org. Chem.*, **12**, 551 (1947).
19. L. H. Briggs, *J. Soc. Chem. Ind.*, **56**, 137 (1937).
20. C. W. Brandt, *N.Z. J. Sci. and Technol.*, **20**, 88 (1938).
21. E. G. Brooker, *N.Z. J. Sci. and Technol.*, **41**, 212 (1959).
22. L. H. Briggs and M. D. Sutherland, *J. Org. Chem.*, **13**, 1 (1948).
23. L. H. Briggs, *J. Soc. Chem. Ind.*, **60**, 222 (1941).
24. L. H. Briggs and W. I. Taylor, *J. Soc. Chem. Ind.*, **66**, 168 (1947).
25. L. H. Briggs and M. D. Sutherland, *J. Org. Chem.*, **7**, 397 (1942).
26. K. Nishida and H. Uota, *J. Agric. Chem. Soc.* (Japan), **11**, 489 (1935).
27. K. Nishida and H. Uota, *J. Agric. Chem. Soc.* (Japan), **12**, 308 (1936).
28. L. H. Briggs, *J. Chem. Soc.*, 1035 (1937).
29. L. H. Briggs, R. C. Cambie, P. S. Rutledge, and D. W. Stanton, *J. Chem. Soc.*, 6212 (1965).
30. C. W. Brandt, *N.Z. J. Sci. and Technol.*, **34**, 36 (1952).
31. C. W. Bottomley, A. R. H. Cole and D. E. White, *J. Chem. Soc.*, 2624 (1655).
32. L. H. Briggs, B. F. Cain, R. C. Cambie and B. R. Davis, *J. Chem. Soc.*, 1840 (1962).
33. L. H. Briggs, *J. N.Z. Inst. Chem.*, **23**, 92 (1959).
34. L. H. Briggs, B. F. Cain, B. R. Davis and J. K. Wilmshurst, *Tetrahedron Letters*, No. 8, 8 et seq. (1959).

35. P. K. GRANT and R. HODGES, *Tetrahedron*, **8**, 261 (1960).
36. J. R. HOSKING, *Ber.*, **69**, 760 (1936).
37. P. K. GRANT and R. HODGES, *J. Chem. Soc.*, 5274 (1960).
38. J. A. BARLTROP and N. A. J. ROGERS, *Chem. and Ind.*, 20 (1957); *J. Chem. Soc.*, 2566 (1958).
39. R. B. TURNER and P. E. SHAW, *Tetrahedron Letters*, No. 18, 24 (1960).
40. R. F. CHURCH, R. E. IRELAND and J. A. MARSHALL, *Tetrahedron Letters*, No. 17, 1 (1960).
41. J. A. BARLTROP, D. GILES, J. R. HANSON, and N. A. J. ROGERS, *J. Chem. Soc.*, 2534 (1962).
42. C. DJERASSI, M. CAIS and C. A. MITSCHER, *J. Amer. Chem. Soc.*, **81**, 2386 (1959).
43. B. E. CROSS, J. R. HANSON, L. H. BRIGGS, R. C. CAMBIE, and P. S. RUTLEDGE, *Proc. Chem. Soc.*, 17 (1963).
44. J. R. HANSON, *J. Chem. Soc.*, 5061 (1963).
45. R. HENDERSON and R. HODGES, *Tetrahedron*, **11**, 226 (1960).
46. L. H. BRIGGS, R. C. CAMBIE and P. S. RUTLEDGE, *J. Chem. Soc.*, 5374 (1963).
47. L. H. BRIGGS, B. F. CAIN, and B. R. DAVIS, *Tetrahedron Letters*, No. 17, 9 (1960).
48. L. H. BRIGGS, B. F. CAIN, R. C. CAMBIE, R. R. DAVIS, and P. S. RUTLEDGE, *J. Chem. Soc.*, 1850 (1962).
49. T. KONDO, H. IMMAURA and M. SUDA, *Bull. Agric. Chem. Soc.* (Japan), **24**, 65 (1960).
50. J. M. BUTLER and J. T. HOLLOWAY, *J. Soc. Chem. and Ind.*, **58**, 233 (1939).
51. J. R. HOSKING, *Rec. Trav. Chim.*, **47**, 578 (1928); **49**, 1036 (1930).
52. L. H. BRIGGS and W. I. TAYLOR, *J. Chem. Soc.*, 407 (1950).
53. B. E. CROSS, R. H. B. GALT, J. R. HANSON, P. J. CURTIS, J. F. GROVE and A. MORRISON, *J. Chem. Soc.*, 2937 (1963).
54. B. E. CROSS, R. H. B. GALT, and J. R. HANSON, *J. Chem. Soc.*, 295 (1964).
55. S. UCHIDA, *J. Amer. Chem. Soc.*, **38**, 687 (1916).
56. L. H. BRIGGS, B. F. CAIN, R. C. CAMBIE, B. R. DAVIS, P. S. RUTLEDGE, and J. K. WILMSHURST, *J. Chem. Soc.*, 1345 (1963).
57. B. E. CROSS, R. H. B. GALT, J. R. HANSON, and W. KLYNE, *Tetrahedron Letters*, 145 (1962).
58. C. DJERASSI, P. QUITT, E. MOSETTIG, R. C. CAMBIE, P. S. RUTLEDGE, and L. H. BRIGGS, *J. Amer. Chem. Soc.*, **83**, 3720 (1961).
59. E. MOSETTIG, U. BEGLINGER, F. DOLDER, H. LICHTI, P. QUITT, and J. A. WATERS, *J. Amer. Chem. Soc.*, **85**, 2305 (1963).
60. H. VORBRUEGGEN and C. DJERASSI, *Tetrahedron Letters*, 119 (1961).
61. H. VORBRUEGGEN and C. DJERASSI, *J. Amer. Chem. Soc.*, **84**, 2990 (1962).
62. B. E. CROSS, R. H. B. GALT, and J. R. HANSON, *J. Chem. Soc.*, 2944 (1963).
63. B. E. CROSS, R. H. B. GALT, and J. R. HANSON, *J. Chem. Soc.*, 3783 (1963).
64. P. F. SOMMER, V. P. ARYA and W. SIMON, *Tetrahedron Letters*, **20**, 18 (1960).
65. J. R. HANSON, *Tetrahedron*, **22**, 1701 (1966).
66. R. H. B. GALT and J. R. HANSON, *J. Chem. Soc.*, 1565 (1965).
67. B. E. CROSS and K. NORTON, *J. Chem. Soc.*, 1570 (1965).
68. J. R. HANSON, *Tetrahedron*, **22**, 2877 (1966).
69. J. R. HANSON, *Tetrahedron*, **22**, 1453 (1966).
70. J. R. HANSON, *Tetrahedron*, **23**, 801 (1967).
71. M. BARNES and J. MACMILLAN, *J. Chem. Soc.*, 361 (1967).
72. E. WENKERT, *Chem. and Ind.*, 282 (1955).
73. A. J. MCALEES, R. MCCRINDLE, and R. D. H. MURRAY, *Chem. and Ind.*, 240 (1966); *J. Chem. Soc.* (C), 2319 (1966); R. A. APPLETON and A. MCCORMICK, *Tetrahedron*, **24**, 633 (1968).
74. A. H. KAPADI and SUKH DEV, *Tetrahedron Letters*, 1255 (1965); J. R. HANSON, *Tetrahedron*, **23**, 793 (1967); A. YOSHIKOSHI, M. KITADANI and Y. KITAHARA, *Tetrahedron*, **23**, 1175 (1967).
75. E. L. GHISALBERTI and P. R. JEFFERIES, *Aust. J. Chem.*, **19**, 1759 (1966).
76. G. HUGEL, L. LODS, J. M. MELLOR. G. OURISSON, *Bull Soc. Chem.*, 2894 (1965).

77. G. HUGEL, L. LODS, J. M. MELLOR, D. W. THEOBALD, and G. OURISSON, *Bull. Soc. Chem.*, 2882 (1965).
78. C. A. HENRICK and P. R. JEFFERIES, *Chem. and Ind.*, 1801 (1963); *Aust. J. Chem.*, **17**, 578 (1964).
79. B. D. CAVELL and J. MACMILLAN, *Phytochemistry*. **6**, 1107 (1967).
80. R. H. B. GALT and J. R. HANSON, *Chem. and Ind.*, 837 (1964); *Tetrahedron*, **22**, 3185 (1966).
81. M. KATSUMI, B. O. PHINNEY, P. R. JEFFERIES and C. A. HENRICK, *Science*, **144**, 849 (1964).
82. C. A. HENRICK and P. R. JEFFERIES, *Tetrahedron Letters*, 1507 (1964).
83. G. V. BADDELEY, M. W. JARVIS, P. R. JEFFERIES, and R. S. ROSICH, *Aust. J. Chem.*, **17**, 578 (1964).
84. A. GAUDEMER, J. POLONSKY, and E. WENKERT, *Bull. Soc. Chim.*, 407 (1964).
85. G. V. BADDELEY, P. R. JEFFERIES, and R. W. RETALLACK, *Tetrahedron*, **20**, 1983 (1964).
86. M. BRIDEL and R. LAVIEILLE, *Compt. Rend.*, **192**, 1123 (1931).
87. F. BELL, *Chem. and Ind.*, 897 (1954).
88. H. B. WOOD, R. ALLERTON, K. W. DIEHL, H. G. FLETCHER, *J. Org. Chem.*, **20**, 875 (1955).
89. E. VIS and H. G. FLETCHER, *J. Amer. Chem. Soc.*, **78**, 4709 (1956).
90. E. MOSETTIG and W. R. NES, *J. Org. Chem.*, **20**, 884 (1955).
91. F. DOLDER, H. LICHTI, E. MOSETTIG, and P. QUITT, *J. Amer. Chem. Soc.*, **82**, 246 (1960).
92. E. MOSETTIG, P. QUITT, U. BEGLINGER, J. A. WATERS, H. VORBRUEGGEN, and C. DJERASSI, *J. Amer. Chem. Soc.*, **83**, 3163 (1961).
93. J. A. WATERS, E. D. BECKER, and E. MOSETTIG, *J. Org. Chem.*, **27**, 4689 (1962).
94. G. HUGEL, L. LODS, J. M. MELLOR, D. W. THEOBALD, and G. OURISSON, *Bull. Soc. Chim.*, 2888 (1964).
95. R. O. BENGIS and R. J. ANDERSON, *J. Biol. Chem.*, **97**, 99 (1932).
96. K. H. SLOTTA and K. NEISSER, *Ber.*, **71**, 1991, 2342 (1938).
97. K. HAUPTMANN and J. FRANCA, *Z. Physiol. Chem.*, **259**, 245 (1939); *J. Amer. Chem. Soc.*, **65**, 81 (1943).
98. K. HAUPTMANN, J. FRANCA, and L. BRUICK-LACERDA, *J. Amer. Chem. Soc.*, **65**, 993 (1943).
99. A. WETTSTEIN, H. FRITZSCHE, F. HUNZICKER, and K. MIESCHER, *Helv. Chim. Acta*, **24**, 332E (1941).
100. A. WETTSTEIN and K. MIESCHER, *Helv. Chim. Acta*, **25**, 718 (1942).
101. C. DJERASSI, E. WILFRED, L. VISCO and A. J. LEMIN, *J. Org. Chem.*, **18**, 1449 (1953).
102. A. WETTSTEIN and K. MIESCHER, *Helv. Chim. Acta*, **26**, 631 (1943).
103. A. WETTSTEIN and K. MIESCHER, *Helv. Chim. Acta*, **26**, 788 (1943).
104. A. WETTSTEIN, F. HUNZICKER, and K. MIESCHER, *Helv. Chim. Acta*, **26**, 1197 (1943).
105. P. N. CHAKROVORTY and M. M. WESNER, *J. Amer. Chem. Soc.*, **64**, 2235 (1942).
106. P. N. CHAKROVORTY, M. M. WESNER, and R. H. LEVIN, *J. Amer. Chem. Soc.*, **65**, 929 (1943).
107. P. N. CHAKROVORTY, M. M. WESNER, R. H. LEVIN, and G. REED, *J. Amer. Chem. Soc.*, **65**, 1325 (1943).
108. C. DJERASSI, H. BENDAS, and P. SENGUPTA, *J. Org. Chem.*, **20**, 1046 (1955).
109. R. D. HAWORTH, A. H. JUBB, and J. MCKENNA, *J. Chem. Soc.*, 1983 (1955).
110. R. D. HAWORTH and R. A. W. JOHNSTONE, *Chem. and Ind.*, 168 (1956); *J. Chem. Soc.*, 1492 (1957).
111. H. BENDAS and C. DJERASSI, *Chem. and Ind.*, 1481 (1955).
112. C. DJERASSI, M. CAIS, and L. A. MITSCHER, *J. Amer. Chem. Soc.*, **80**, 247 (1958).
113. C. DJERASSI and R. A. FINNEGAN, *J. Amer. Chem. Soc.*, **82**, 4342 (1960).
114. A. I. SCOTT, G. A. SIM, G. FERGUSON, D. W. YOUNG, and F. MCCAPRA, *J. Amer. Chem. Soc.*, **84**, 3197 (1962); A. I. SCOTT, F. MCCAPRA, F. COMER, S. A. SUTHERLAND, D. W. YOUNG, G. A. SIM, and G. FERGUSON, *Tetrahedron*, **20**, 1339 (1964).
115. R. A. FINNEGAN, *J. Org. Chem.*, **26**, 3057 (1961).

116. D. H. R. BARTON, *Quart. Rev.*, **3**, 36 (1949).
117. H. P. KAUFMANN and A. K. SEN GUPTA, *Ber.*, **96**, 2489 (1963).
118. M. C. PEREZAMADOR and F. GARCIA JIMENEZ, *Tetrahedron*, **22**, 1937 (1966); M. C. PEREZAMADOR, F. GARCIA JIMENEZ, J. HERRAN and S. E. FLORES, *Tetrahedron*, **20**, 2999 (1964).
119. T. AJELLO, F. PIOZZI, A. QUILICO, and V. SPRIO, *Rend. Accad. Lincei*, **28**, 454 (1960); *Gazz. Chim. Ital.*, **94**, 867 (1963); F. PIOZZI, A. QUILICO, T. AJELLO, V. SPRIO, A. MELERA, *Tetrahedron Letters*, 1829 (1965).
120. B. E. CROSS, R. H. B. GALT, and J, R. HANSON, *J. Chem. Soc.*, 5052 (1963).
121. R. H. B. GALT and J. R. HANSON, *J. Chem. Soc.*, 1565 (1965).
122. M. TAKAHASHI, T. FUJITA, and Y. KOYAMA, *J. Pharm. Soc.* (Japan), **78**, 699 (1958); **80**, 594, 696 (1960).
123. T. KUBOTA, T. MATSURA, T. TSUTSUI, and K. NAYA, *Bull. Chem. Soc.* (Japan), **34**, 1737 (1961).
124. T. KUBOTA, T. MATSURA, T. TSUTSUI, S. UYEO, M. TAKAHASHI, H. IRIE, A. NUMATA, T. FUJITA, T. OKAMOTO, M. NATSUME, Y. KAWAZOE, K. SUDO, T. IKEDA, M. TOMOEDA, S. KANATOMO, T. KOSUKI, and K. ADOCKI, *Tetrahedron Letters*, 1243 (1964); *Tetrahedron*, **22**, 1659 (1966).
125. Y. LITAKA and M. NATSUME, *Tetrahedron Letters*, 1257 (1964).
126. K. SHUDO, M. NATSUME, and T. OKAMOTO, *Chem. and Pharm. Bull.*, 1019 (1965); *Chem. Comm.*, 468 (1967).
127. E. FUJITA, T. FUJITA, K. FUJI, and N. ITO, *Chem. and Pharm. Bull.*, 1023 (1965); *Chem. Comm.*, 148, 252 (1967); T. KUBOTA and I. KUBO, *Tetrahedron Letters*, 3781 (1967).
128. E. FUJITA, T. FUJITA, and M. SHIBUYA, *Tetrahedron Letters*, 3153 (1966).
129. Cf. A. A. FORSYTH, *British Poisonous Plants*, H.M. Stationery Office, 1954.
130. H. B. WOOD, V. L. STROMBERG, J. C. KERESZETSKY, and E. C. HORNING, *J. Amer. Chem. Soc.*, **76**, 5689 (1954).
131. T. TAKEMOTO and H. MEGURI, *J. Pharm. Chem.* (Japan), **29**, 588 (1957).
132. W. H. TALLENT, M. C. REITHOF and E. C. HORNING, *J. Amer. Chem. Soc.*, **79**, 4548 (1957).
133. S. W. HARDIKER, *K. Pharmacol. Exper. Therap.*, **20**, 17 (1922); N. C. NORAN, P. E. DRESEL, M. E. PERKINS, and A. P. RICHARDSON, *J. Pharmacol. Exper. Therap.*, **110**, 415 (1954).
134. H. KAKISAWA, M. KURONO, S. TAKAHASHI, and Y. HIRATA, *Tetrahedron Letters*, 59 (1961).
135. J. IWASA, Z. KUMAZAWA and M. NAKAJIMA, *Chem. and Ind.*, 511 (1961).
136. H. KAKISAWA, *J. Chem. Soc.* (Japan), **82**, 1096, 1216 (1961).
137. H. KAKISAWA, M. YANAI, T. KOZIMA, K. NAKANISHI, and H. MISHIMA, *Tetrahedron Letters*, 215 (1962).
138. W. TALLENT, *J. Org. Chem.*, **27**, 2968 (1962); **29**, 2756 (1964).
139. T. KOZIMA, K. NAKANISHI, M. YANAI, and H. KAKISAWA, *Tetrahedron Letters*, 1329 (1964); *Tetrahedron* **21**, 3091 (1965).
140. H. A. LLOYD and H. M. FALES, *Tetrahedron Letters*, 4891 (1967).
141. P. COATES, A. K. GOH, P. R. JEFFERIES, J. R. KNOX and T. G. PAYNE, *Tetrahedron*, **24**, 795 (1968).
142. D. A. H. TAYLOR, *J. Chem. Soc.* (C), 1360 (1967).
143. J. R. CHANNON, P. W. CHOW, P. R. JEFFERIES and G. V. MEEHAN, *Aust. J. Chem.*, **19**, 861 (1966).
144. D. E. EKONG and A. U. OGAN, *J. Chem. Soc.* (C), 311 (1968).
145. E. L. GHISALBERTI, P. R. JEFFERIES and W. A. MINCHAM, *Tetrahedron*, **23**, 4463 (1967).
146. E. L. GHISALBERTI, P. R. JEFFERIES, S. PASSANNANTI and F. PIOZZI, *Aust. J. Chem.*, **21**, 459 (1968).
147. J. R. HANSON and A. F. WHITE, *Tetrahedron*, **24**, 2533 (1968).
148. J. R. HANSON and A. F. WHITE, *Tetrahedron*, **24**, 2527 (1968).
149. E. FUJITA, T. FUJITA and H. KATAYAMA, *Chem. Comm.*, 968 (1967).

CHAPTER 3

THE GIBBERELLINS

3.1. *Introduction*

The culture filtrate of some strains of the fungus *Gibberella fujikuroi*—the causative organism of the bakanae disease of rice seedlings—contains a group of metabolites known as the gibberellins. The earlier work on these was limited almost exclusively to Japan and culminated in 1938[1,2] in the isolation of an active metabolite with powerful growth-promoting properties. However, it was hampered by the fact that this so-called gibberellin A was a mixture of closely related compounds. Gibberellic acid, which is the best known of the gibberellins, was isolated[3] from the ACC 917 strain at the Akers Research Laboratories of I.C.I. in the early 1950's. This metabolite affected many aspects of normal plant growth and development. Subsequently small amounts of related gibberellins have been isolated from higher plants and are regarded as natural plant growth hormones. The chemical[4,5] and biological[6–11] properties of these compounds have been the subject of several reviews, whilst a procedure has been proposed[100] for the allocation of trivial names to new gibberellins.

Gibberellic acid, $C_{19}H_{22}O_6$ (I), was characterized[12] as a tetracarbocyclic dihydroxy-γ-lactonic acid containing two ethylenic bonds. It gave a methyl ester and a mono- and di-acetate whilst the presence of a γ-lactone was indicated by the infrared spectrum of a number of derivatives which showed characteristic absorption in the range 1765–1770 cm.$^{-1}$ The acid consumed two equivalents of alkali on titration. Insight into the structure of gibberellic acid was obtained by studying the products of acidic degradation. Mild acid hydrolysis afforded an aromatic hydroxy-acid, allogibberic acid (gibberellin B[13,14]) $C_{18}H_{22}O_3$ (II), and carbon dioxide. The acid was isomerized under more vigorous conditions to a second aromatic acid, gibberic acid (III). On dehydrogenation gibberellic acid, allogibberic acid and gibberic acid all gave a hydrocarbon, gibberene[14] shown by synthesis[15] to be 1,7-dimethylfluorene (IV) thus revealing the unique carbon skeleton of the gibberellins.

3.2. *The Structure of Gibberic Acid*

The oxidative degradation[16,17] of gibberic acid led to the structure (III). Thus oxidation with selenium dioxide gave an α-diketone, gibberdionic acid[12, 18] (V) indicating the presence of a methylene α- to the carbonyl group. This diketone was not enolizable and hence the carbonyl groups must be attached to quaternary or bridgehead positions. Cleavage of the dione with alkaline hydrogen peroxide followed by dehydrogenation still gave 1,7-dimethylfluorene and hence dehydrogenation is accompanied by elimination of the methylene carbonyl bridge. The position of the carboxyl group in gibberic acid was established by relatively mild dehydrogenation of methyl gibberdionate to 9-methoxycarbonyl-1,7-dimethylfluorene. Vigorous oxidation of gibberic acid gave benzene-1, 2,3-tricarboxylic acid indicating the substitution pattern of the benzenoid ring. The position of the methylene carbonyl group on the fluorene skeleton was determined by oxidation of gibberic acid with alkaline potassium permanganate. This gave dehydrogibberic acid which on decarboxylation with palladium charcoal formed gibberone (VI). Ultraviolet spectra showed that the new double bond was in conjugation with the aromatic ring. The ethylenic bond in gibberone was then cleaved with chromic oxide to give a mono-basic keto-acid (VII) which from its spectral characteristics and further behaviour on oxidation contained both a 2,2-disubstituted indan-1-one and a cyclopentanone. Proof of the structure of this keto-acid was obtained by opening both non-benzenoid rings and synthesizing[19] the product (VIII). Thus the cyclopentanone (VII) was

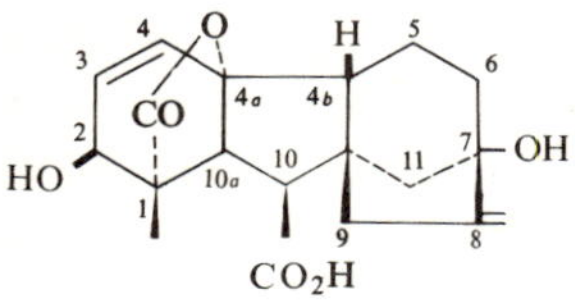

I

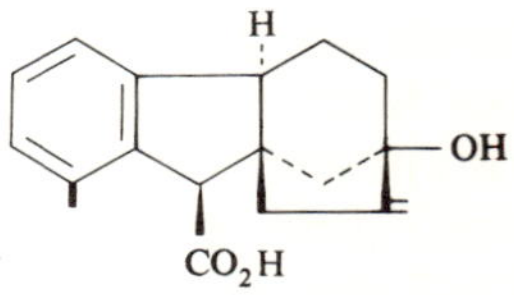

II

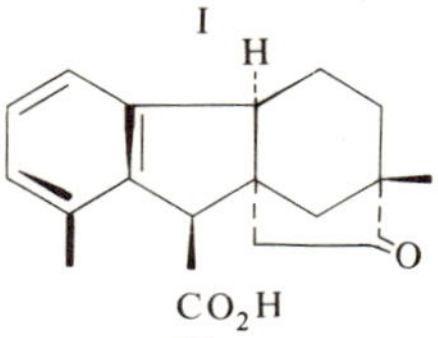

III

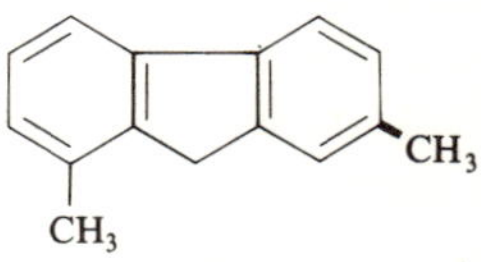

IV

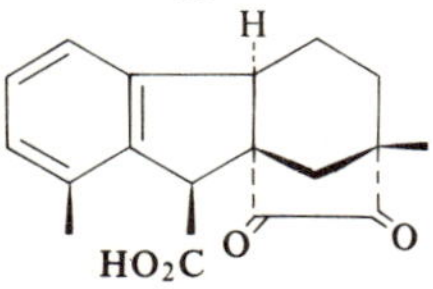

V

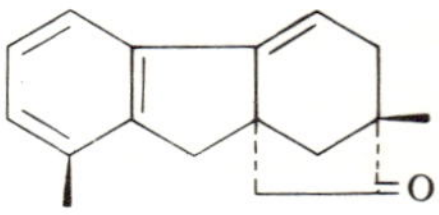

VI

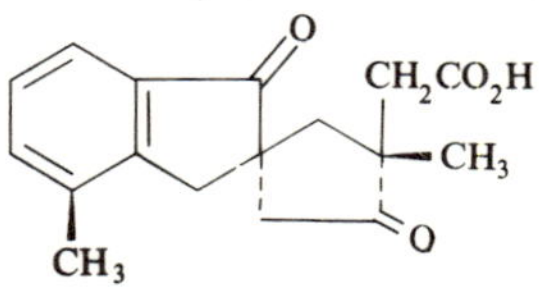

VII

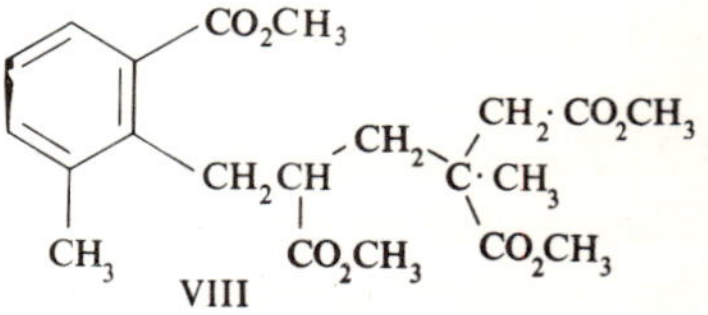

VIII

converted to an α-hydroxyimino ketone which on Beckmann rearrangement with toluene-*p*-sulphonyl chloride followed by alkaline hydrolysis gave a cyanotricarboxylic acid. This was further hydrolysed by sulphuric acid to a mixture of diastereo-isomeric tetracarboxylic acids (VIII) purified as their methyl esters. These were then synthesized.

3.3. *The Structure of Allogibberic Acid*

Allogibberic acid (II) contained, in place of the cyclopentanone of gibberic acid, an ethylenic double bond and a hydroxyl group. The latter resisted oxidation and was therefore tertiary. Indeed when dihydroallogibberic acid was oxidized with alkaline potassium permanganate, a dehydro derivative was formed in which an ethylenic double bond was introduced in conjugation with the benzene ring. Ozonolysis of allogibberic acid gave formaldehyde and an α-ketol (IX) which was in turn

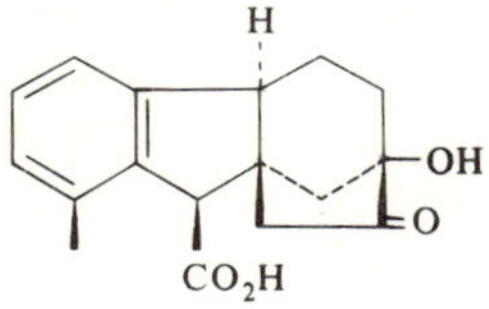

IX 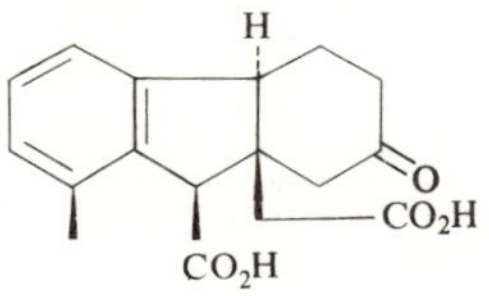 X

oxidized to a dibasic keto-acid (X). The infrared spectrum of this ketol indicated that it formed part of a cyclopentanone. The dibasic keto-acid readily formed an anhydride with the 9-carboxyl from which it was recovered on hydrolysis. The position of the hydroxyl group of allogibberic acid and one point of attachment of the five-membered ring on the hexahydrofluorene skeleton were then established by dehydrogenation of both the dibasic keto-acid (X) and dihydroallogibberic acid to 8-methylfluoren-2-ol. In this dehydrogenation all the non-skeletal carbon atoms except the aromatic methyl group were eliminated and hence the second point of attachment of ring D must be angular. Of these positions only 8a permitted the formation of dehydro derivatives conjugated with the aromatic ring and of an internal anhydride between the two carboxyls of the dibasic acid (X). It followed that allogibberic acid had the structure (II) allowing a Wagner–Meerwein rearrangement to gibberic acid (III).[21]

In a feature which is typical of gibberellin chemistry 4b epimers of these acids were known.[22] Gibberellenic acid (XI) which was formed[23–25] from the aqueous decomposition of gibberellic acid or by treatment with hydrazine hydrate at 150° gave on mild acid hydrolysis, allogibberic acid and an isomer shown to be its 4b-epimer, 4b-epiallogibberic acid (XII). The action of hot mineral acid on gibberellic acid gave both gibberic acid and 4b-epigibberic acid (XIII). The relationship between these and the relative configuration of their asymmetric centres were assigned[22] on the following basis.

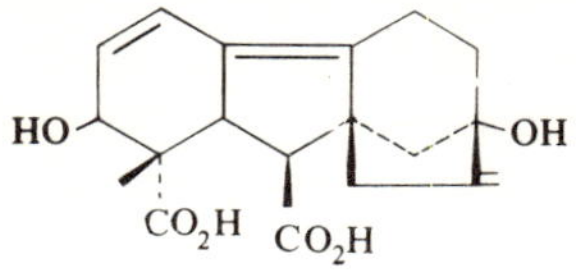

XI 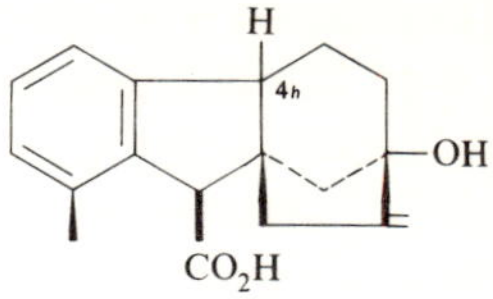 XII

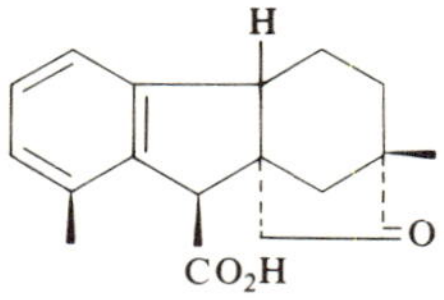

XIII 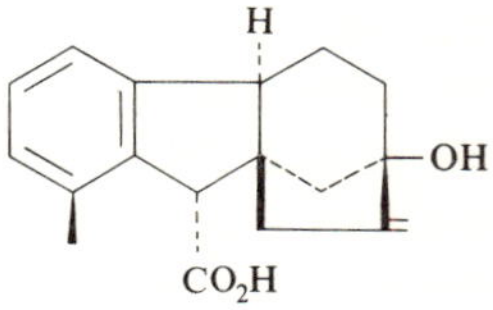 XIV

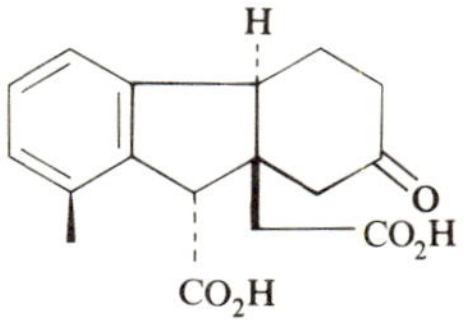

XV 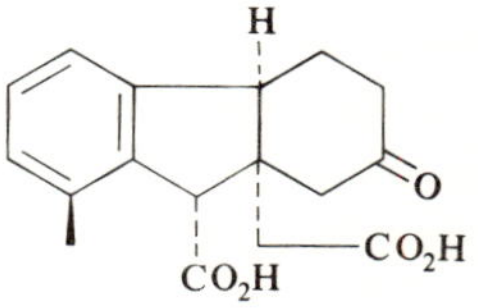 XVI

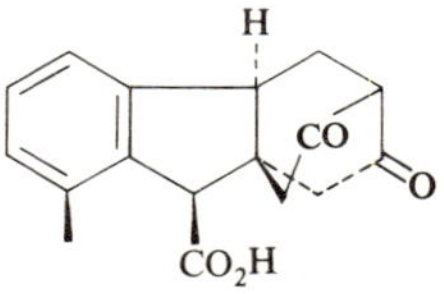

XVII 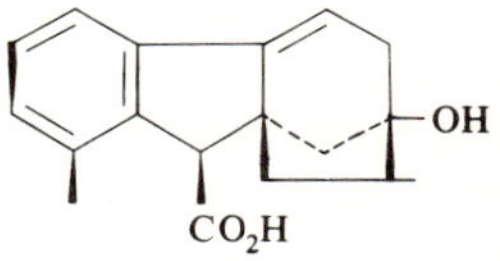 XVIII

Ozonolysis of allogibberic acid led to the ketol (IX) and the dibasic keto-acid (X). During this work six of the possible eight stereoisomers (X) were isolated. Thus alkaline hydrolysis of both methyl allogibberate and the half-ester obtained by ozonolysis of methyl allogibberate gave predominantly the 9α-acids (XV) and (XVI). However, alkaline hydrolysis of the dimethyl ester of (X) led not only to epimerization at 9 but also to inversion of the acetic acid side-chain to form *inter alia* (XVI). The intermediate 1:3-diketone (XVIII) arising by an intramolecular Claisen condensation has been isolated[26] by the reaction of acetic anhydride with the keto-acid (X). The isolation of compounds of this type has been found in the kaurene series. No inversion of this side chain occurred in the 4b-epiallogibberic acid series. Furthermore, isomerization led to more equal amounts of 9 epimers. Anhydrides were readily and reversibly formed between the carboxyl groups of (X) and (XVI) which were therefore *cis* to one another thus establishing the relative configuration of ring D and the carboxyl group. Evidence for the stereochemistry of the B/C fusion came from hydrogenation experiments. Hydrogenation of 4b-dehydro-dihydroallogibberic acid (XVIII) regenerated dihydroallogibberic acid and since reduction is likely to occur from the less-hindered (α) face of the molecule, rings B and C of allogibberic acid are *trans* fused and *cis* fused in 4b-epiallogibberic acid.

Evidence[22,27] for the absolute stereochemistry of these degradation products came from the positive Cotton effect in the optical rotatory dispersion curve of the dimethyl ester of (X), which was compared[28] with model hexahydroindanones of known absolute stereochemistry. Further studies[29] revealed the influence of the stereochemistry at position 9 on the sign of the plain curve upon which the Cotton effects are superimposed. The mechanism of the Wagner–Meerwein rearrangement requires the two-carbon bridge of gibberic acid to have the opposite configuration to that of allogibberic acid. This was supported by optical rotatory dispersion measurements on the corresponding ketones.

3.4. *The Structure of Gibberellic Acid*

These results were then extended[30,31] to provide evidence for the complete structure of gibberellic acid. Since methyl gibberellate gave methyl gibberate on treatment with mineral acid the 10-carboxyl group was common to both. In the formation of allogibberic acid from gibberellic acid, aromatization of ring A was accompanied by the loss of a hydroxyl group and the γ-lactone ring. Ring A of gibberellic acid therefore contains[32] a double bond, a saturated γ-lactone and a hydroxyl group. This hydroxyl group was shown to be secondary by oxidation of methyl tetrahydrogibberellate to a monohydroxy ketone. Despite earlier evidence to the contrary,[30] oxidation of methyl gibberellate with manganese dioxide gave[31] an $\alpha\beta$-unsaturated ketone (λ_{max}228mμ log ϵ 3·99) having the substitution O=C · CH=CH— and hence the secondary hydroxyl group was allylic to the double bond. The location of this hydroxyl group on the carbon skeleton came from the dehydrogenation of the ring A ketone (XIX) (obtained by Wagner–Meerwein isomerization and oxidation of gibberellin A_1) to 1,7-dimethylfluoren-2-ol.[33]

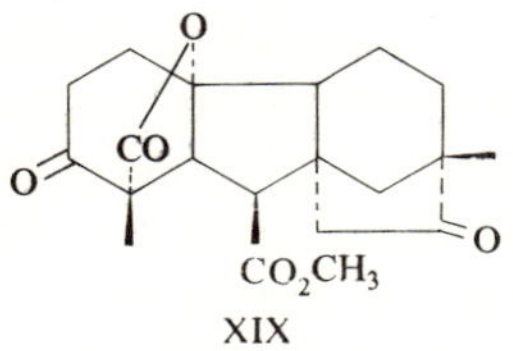

O CO O O CO_2CH_3

XIX

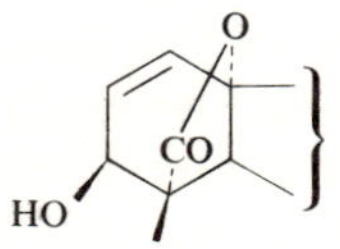

O CO HO

XX

On hydrogenation of the ring A double bond considerable hydrogenolysis of the lactone ring occurred giving 30–70 per cent acidic products depending on the nature of the solvent. Furthermore, the heteroannular dienic dibasic acid, gibberellenic acid (XI) was obtained from the aqueous decomposition of gibberellic acid. This suggested that the oxygen of the γ-lactone in gibberellic acid was allylic to the double bond. This led to the structure (XX) for ring A which in turn received[34,35] support from the nuclear magnetic resonance spectra. In particular in the spectrum of methyl diacetylgibberellate, the methyl group appeared as a singlet (τ 8·86) whilst the C-3 proton appeared as a quartet (τ 4·16) coupled both to the C-4 proton (τ 4·68) and to the C-2 proton (τ 3·62).

3.5. *The Stereochemistry of Gibberellic Acid*

The optical rotatory dispersion curve of the norketone (XXI) showed a positive Cotton effect[29,36] and therefore ring D of the gibberellins and hence the 8a-acetic acid side chain of the seco-acid (XXII) had the β-configuration. The carboxyl groups of this acid reversibly formed an intramolecular anhydride and hence the 10-carboxyl group also had a β-configuration. The magnitude of the coupling constant between the 10 and 10a protons in the nuclear magnetic resonance spectrum was taken as evidence for a *trans*-relationship between these two protons (i.e. a β-10a-proton).

The stereochemistry of ring A and in particular the orientation of the lactone ring was the source of some controversy.[36–39] The optical rotatory dispersion curve of methyl 2-ketotetrahydrogibberellate showed a strong positive Cotton effect similar to that of (+)-homoepicamphor pointing to an α-oriented lactone bridge. Furthermore, hydrogenolysis of the lactone ring took place with inversion at C_{4a}. The ring A ketone (XXIII) then obtained by decarboxylation and oxidation of the hydrogenolysis acid showed a negative Cotton effect which was taken to imply a 10a β-hydrogen and probably a *cis* A/B ring fusion. However, arguments based[37,38] on the molecular rotation differences on opening the lactone ring suggested incorrectly that it was in fact β. Since the base-catalysed epimerization of the 2-hydroxyl in gibberellin A_1 derivatives implied that it possessed an axial configuration the distinction had to be made between the two absolute configurations (XXIV) and (XXV) for ring A. An α-oriented lactone ring required the more stable *trans* A/B ring junction (XXIV) in contrast to the β-oriented lactone ring which required the *cis* fusion (XXV). The former was more consistent with the ready relactonization and rearrangement of a 1–4a lactone to a 1–3 lactone (XXVI) together with the elimination and substitution reactions of the epimeric 2-hydroxyl groups. Thus the equatorial 2-hydroxyl was more readily toluene-*p*-sulphonated and the derived toluene-*p*-sulphonate more stable than the axial derivative to olefin formation. The axial alcohol on reaction with phosphorus pentachloride gave a good yield of the gibb-2-ene whilst the equatorial hydroxyl group underwent substitution. These differences would not be expected from the more strained *cis* fusion. Treatment of gibberellin A_1 methyl ester (XXVII) with 2N-hydrochloric acid gave rise through a 4a carbonium ion to an equilibrium

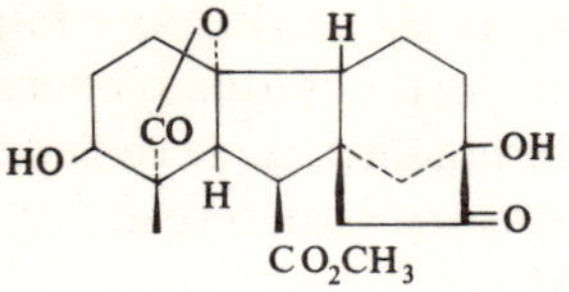

XXI

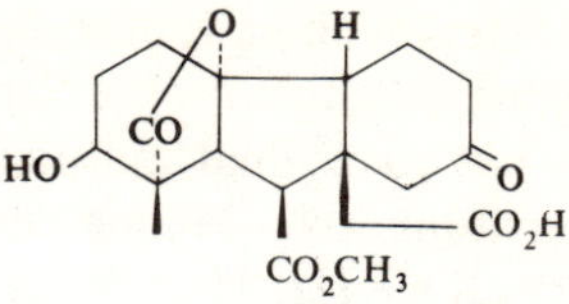

XXII

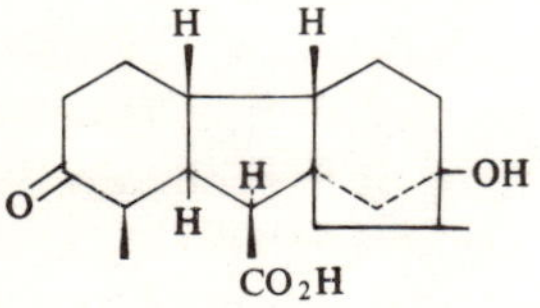

XXIII

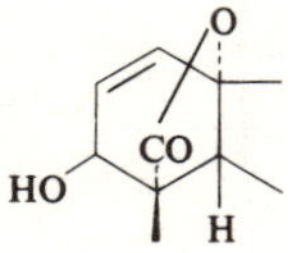

XXIV

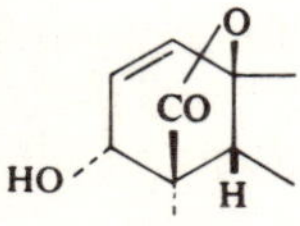

XXV

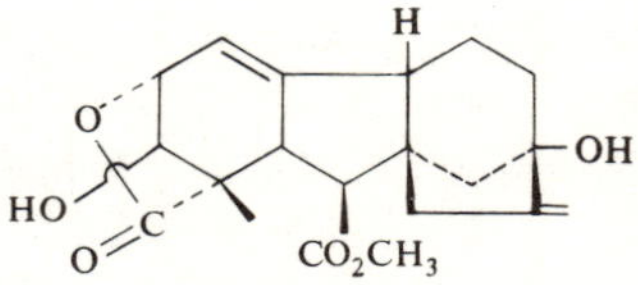

XXVI

mixture of 4b epimers (XXVIII) together with the 4a:4b unsaturated ester (XXIX). Under these conditions although there was incorporation of deuterium from a deuterium chloride experiment there was no inversion at the adjacent 10a suggesting that this was the more stable A/B fusion and hence ring A has the stereochemistry (XXIV). Application of the atrolactic acid method to C-2 lent support to this.

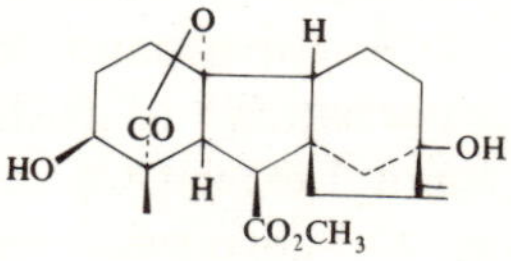

XXVII

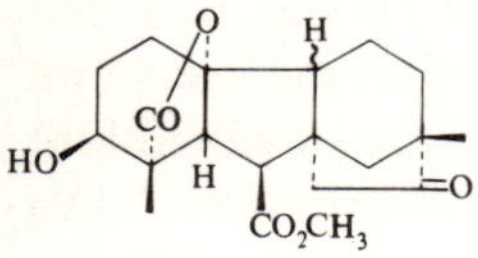

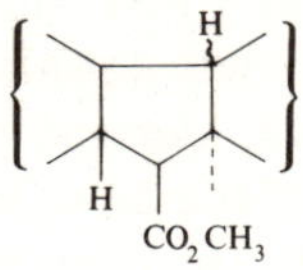

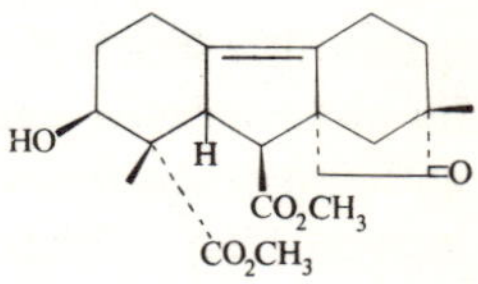

XXVIII

XXIX

The methyl ester of (XXII) showed a positive Cotton effect similar to that of the related compound (X) derived from allogibberic acid and hence gibberellic acid was initially assigned the same B/C/D ring fusion, i.e. a 4bα-hydrogen. However, further optical rotatory dispersion studies by the same group of workers using the plain curves of 4b epimers and a *cis*-fused lactone of the type (XXX) demonstrated the weakness of this analogy. Meanwhile circular dichroism studies of the norketones implied the opposite conclusion.[43,44] X-ray analysis of a methyl bromogibberellate (XXXI) led to a final clarification of the problem and revealed a β-hydrogen atom at 4b. Hence gibberellic acid has the structure and stereochemistry (XXXII).

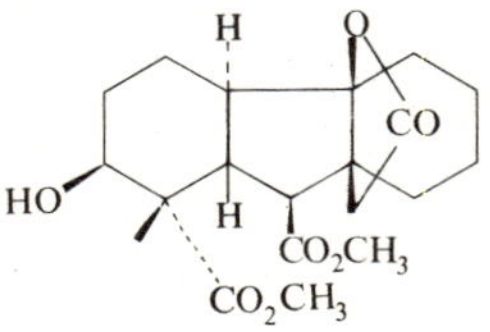

XXX

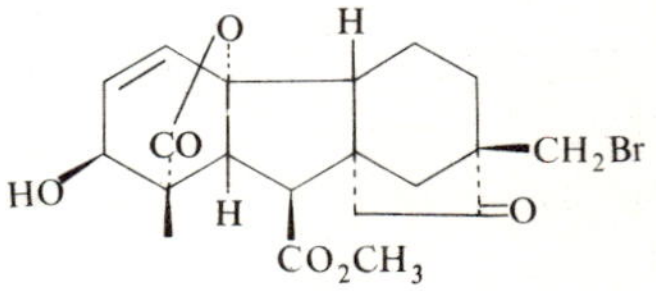

XXXI

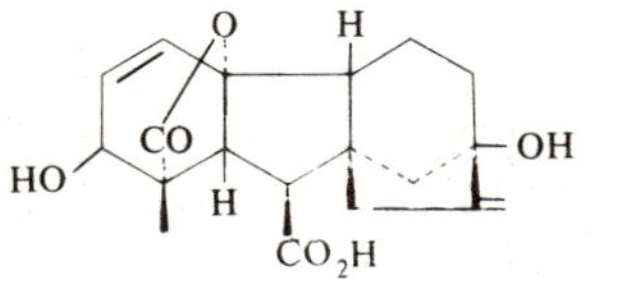

XXXII

3.6. *The Reduction of Gibberellic Acid*

There are two competing reactions in the reduction of the ring A double bond.[45,46] On the one hand this gave gibberellin A_1[47,48] and the 8-epimeric tetrahydro derivatives whilst on the other hand hydrogenolysis led to a mixture of the tetrahydro acids. These, depending on the ease of access of the remaining double bond, could be further reduced to hexahydro acids. Thus the complex nature of acidic products were separated into the 8-epimeric hexahydro acids, the corresponding gibb-4-enes and a gibb-4a(4b)-ene. Controlled hydrogenation[48] of methyl gibberellate (1 mole uptake) gave gibberellin A_1 methyl ester (XXVII) and the hydrogenolysis acid (XXXVI). Ultraviolet end-absorption measurements were used[45] to distinguish between the $\Delta^{4,4a}$ and $\Delta^{4a,4b}$-tetrahydro acids.

Hydrogenolysis brought about inversion at C-4a which was reflected in the difference of reactivity between the hydrogenolysis products and the corresponding gibberellin A_1 derivative. A comparison was therefore made between the reactions of the 2β-(ax)-hydroxy keto-ester (XXXIV) derived from gibberellin A_1 by rearrangement of rings C/D, and the 8-epimethyl ester (XXXV). Toluene-*p*-sulphonation of the 2α-(eq) epimer of (XXXV) took place more readily than with the axial epimer whilst elimination of the axial toluene-*p*-sulphonate with collidine occurred more readily. On the other hand whereas toluene-*p*-sulphonation of the ester (XXXV) occurred readily, its 2-axial epimer was not esterified at that position. On treatment with phosphorus pentachloride the axial hydroxy keto-ester (XXXIV) gave the gibb-2-ene in good yield whilst the equatorial alcohol underwent substitution. In the 8-epi methyl series the results

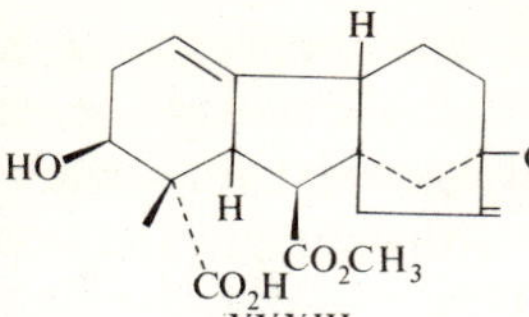

XXXIII

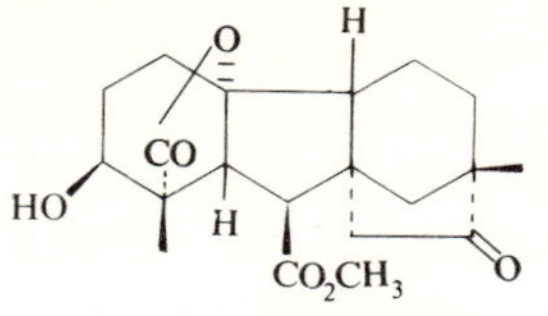

XXXIV

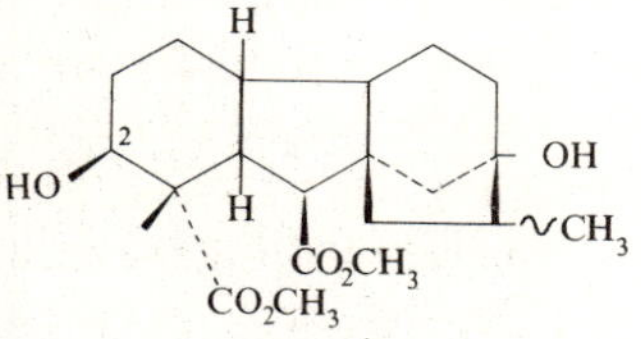

XXXV

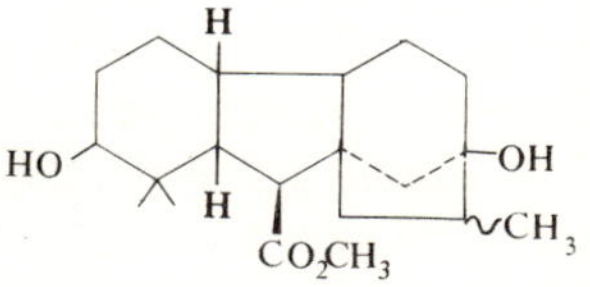

XXXVI

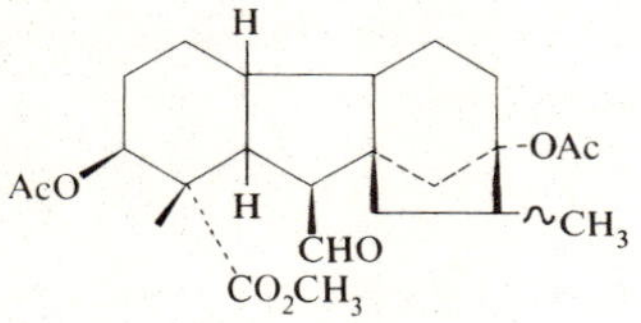

XXXVII

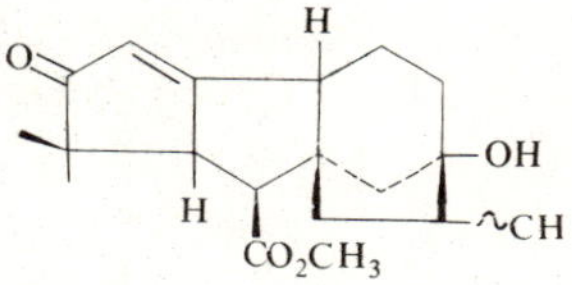

XXXVIII

were less clear cut. The 2β-ester (XXXV) gave mainly substitution products and only a low yield of gibb-2-enes whereas the 2α-epimer, gave only elimination and no substitution products. In contrast to reduction of the gibberellin A_1 2-ketones, sodium borohydride reduction of the 2-ketone corresponding to (XXXV) mainly regenerated the parent alcohol. Furthermore, when the 1-methoxycarbonyl group was converted to a methyl group (XXXVI) elimination of the 2-hydroxyl brought about concomitant ring contraction. Thus this alcohol is now an equatorial substituent on ring A and consequently it was not epimerized by base. In the reduction of the carboxyl group by Rosenmund reduction of the corresponding acid chloride, a 10-aldehyde (XXXVII) was obtained by a by-product – a result which was explained by assuming the intervention of a cyclic oxonium ion which might decompose in either sense. Proof of the *cis* A/B fusion of the hydrogenolysis acids was obtained by conversion of ring A to a cyclopentenone (XXXVIII). In view of the known stability of *cis* and *trans* bicyclo-3,3,0-octanones reduction under equilibrating conditions would be expected to form the *cis* fused product. Indeed reduction with lithium in liquid ammonia regenerated the parent cyclopentane ring system which was therefore *cis* fused.

3.7. *The C-19-Gibberellins*

The structures of the other C_{19} gibberellins were demonstrated by interrelationship with gibberellic acid. Gibberellin A_1 was shown[47] by its preparation from gibberellic acid to be (XXXIX).

Much of the Japanese work was concerned with the structure of gibberellin A_1 for which they initially favoured[49–51] an alternative ring A structure. The major evidence for this rested upon dehydrogenation of the penta-ol derived by lithium aluminium hydride reduction of gibberellin A_1 to a fluorene which they identified as 1:3-dimethylfluorene. However, this was rendered untenable by the relationship with gibberellic acid and by the nuclear magnetic resonance spectra. Dehydration of the Wagner–Meerwein rearrangement product (XXXIV) of gibberellin A_1 gave the 7α-gibbane corresponding to gibberellin A_5[53,54] (XL). This was in turn hydroxylated to establish a relationship with gibberellin A_8 (XLI)[55]. Gibberellin A_6 (XLII) was shown[55] to be an epoxide. Acidic hydrolysis and rearrangement produced a chloro-alcohol. Reductive elimination of halogen then led to (XXXIV). This group of gibberellins were isolated from *Phaseolus multiflorus*.

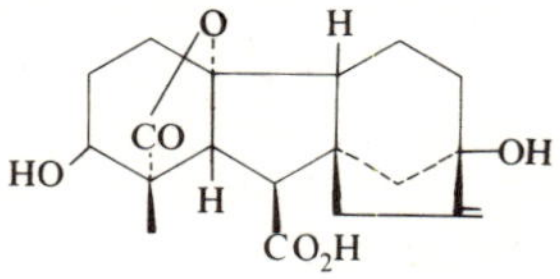

XXXIX

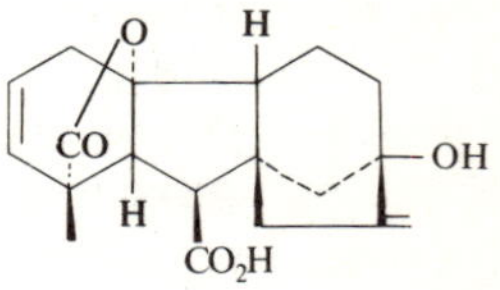

XL

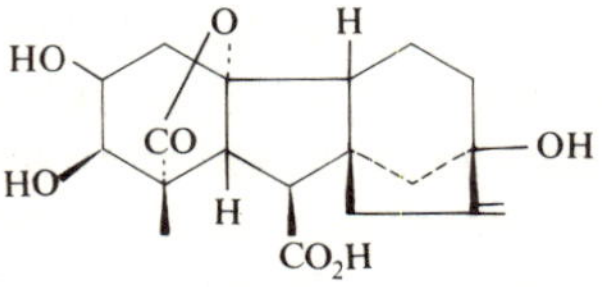

XLI

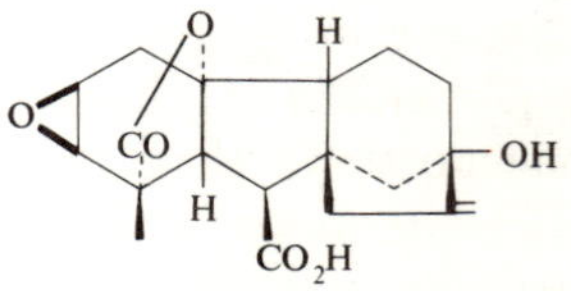

XLII

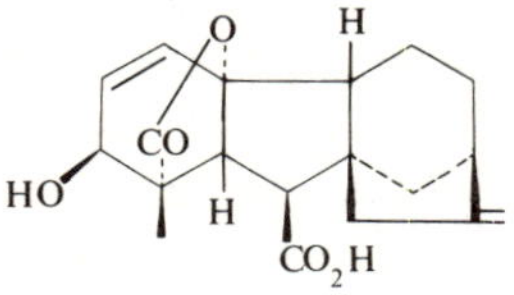

XLIII

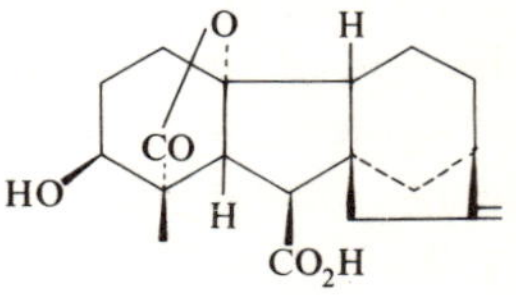

XLIV

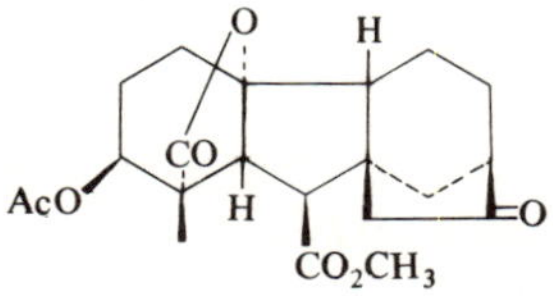

XLV

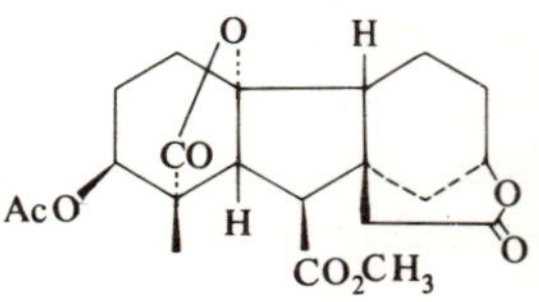

XLVI

The 7-deoxygibberellin, gibberellin A_7 (XLIII) was isolated from a pH adjusted fermentation. It could be reduced to gibberellin A_4 (XLIV). In confirmation of its structure gibberellin A_7 was related to gibberellic acid.

Thus on ozonolysis and reduction it formed a gibberellin A_4 derivative (XLV)[57]. Baeyer–Villiger oxidation of this led[58] to the acetoxy-δ-lactone (XLVI) retaining all the centres of asymmetry of gibberellin A_7. The lactone was also prepared from gibberellic acid. Gibberellin A_7 was shown to have the same ring A chemistry as gibberellic acid. Thus it was oxidized by manganese dioxide and chromium trioxide to an $\alpha\beta$-unsaturated ketone (λ_{max} 228 mμ). On treatment with mineral acid ring A underwent aromatization. Furthermore, the base-catalysed rearrangement to a 1–3 lactone (XLVII) occurred.[59] Selective hydrogenation of the ring A double bond gave gibberellin A_4. Gibberellin A_4 (XLIV) was related to gibberellin A_2 (XLVIII)[60–62] by hydration of the terminal methylene with mineral acid. Gibberellin A_4 (XLIV) was also related by dehydration and hydrogenation to dihydrogibberellin A_9.[63,64] Gibberellin A_{10} (XLIX) was prepared[65] from gibberellin A_9 (L) by hydration with mineral acid whilst gibberellin A_{11} is probably a ring A epoxide. In gibberellin A_{16}[91] the ring A double bond of gibberellin A_7 has been hydrated to give a 4α-alcohol. Gibberellin A_{20} has been identified[92] as the 7-hydroxy derivative of gibberellin A_9 (i.e. dihydrogibberellin A_5). In gibberellin A_{21} (from *Canavalia gladiata*)[93] the 1-methyl group of A_{20} has been oxidized to the level of a carboxylic acid. Gibberellin A_{22} contains the 1-methyl group of gibberellin A_5 at the oxidation level of a primary alcohol.

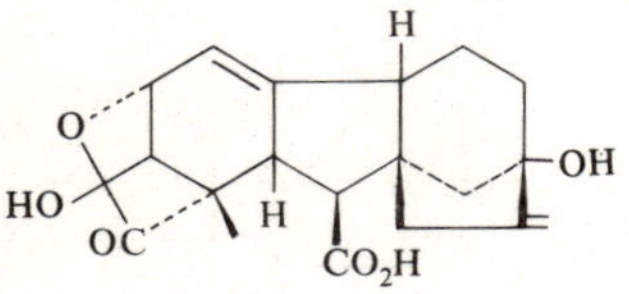

XLVII

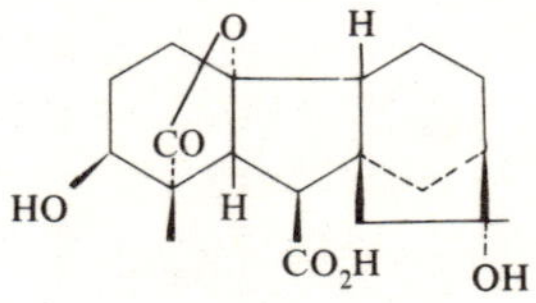

XLVIII

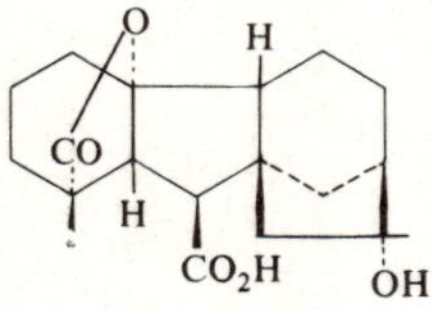

XLIX

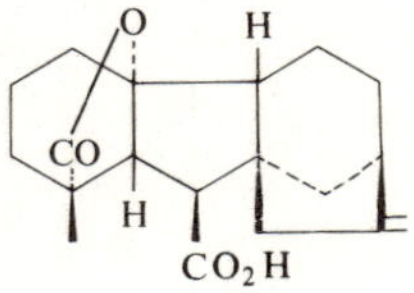

L

3.8. *The Chemistry of the Gibberellins*

The chemistry of the different gibberellins may be distinguished by two features; the presence or absence of the $\Delta^{3,4}$ double bond on the one hand and the 2- and 7-hydroxyls on the other. Thus in the absence of a 7-hydroxyl, the 8-methylene is hydrated by treatment with mineral acid.[62,65] However, the presence of a 7-hydroxyl permits a Wagner–Meerwein rearrangement to the 7α-gibbane system – a rearrangement which may also be brought about by the action of t-butyl hypochlorite,[29] by bromination,[44] and by cleavage of an 8:15 epoxide.[94] Ring A of the gibberellin system is also labile to alkali.[40] In the absence of a $\Delta^{3,4}$ double bond the 2(ax)-hydroxyl of, for example, gibberellin A_1, is epimerized in dilute alkali to an equilibrium mixture containing the 2(eq)-hydroxyl (pseudo-gibberellin A_1). A retroaldol mechanism has been proposed[95] for this. The retro-Claisen reaction of the corresponding ketone has also been observed.[96] In the presence of a $\Delta^{3,4}$ double bond, allylic rearrangement takes place to form a 1–3-lactone (LI) without inversion of the 2(ax)-substituent. Thus gibberellic acid consumed two molecules of dilute alkali at room temperature to form a dicarboxylic acid (LII). The dimethyl ester of this product was cleaved with glycol splitting reagents to give a crystalline lactone (LIII). The structure of this rests upon microhydrogenation and perbenzoic acid determination of the double bonds together with the absence of significant ultraviolet absorption.

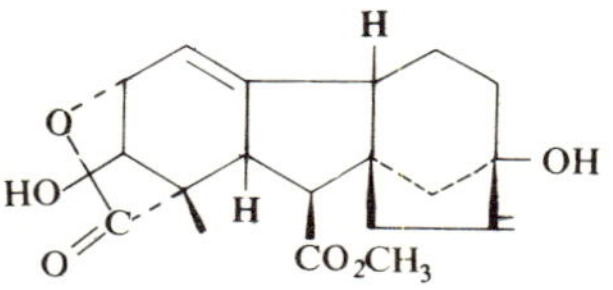

LI

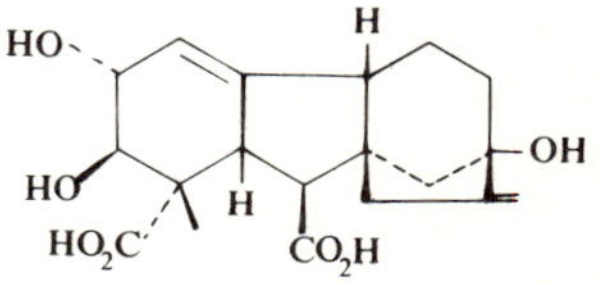

LII

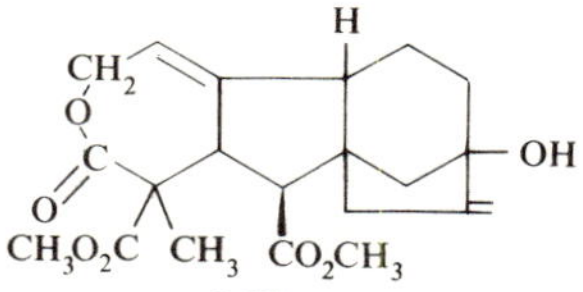

LIII

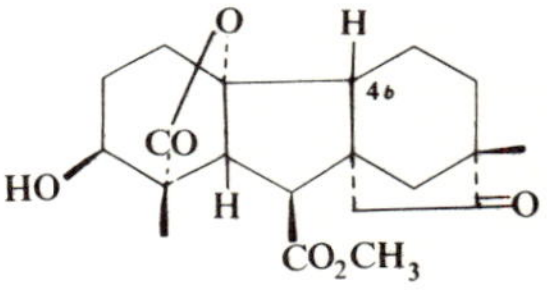

LIV

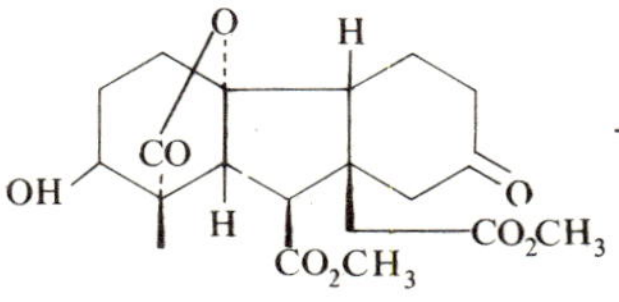

LV

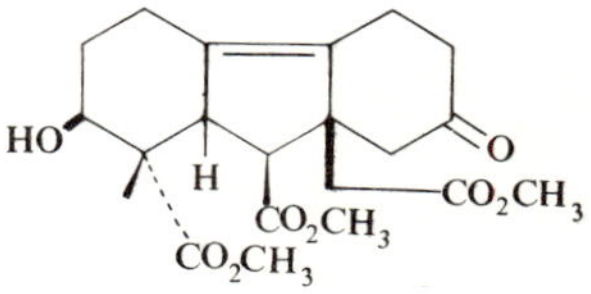

LVI

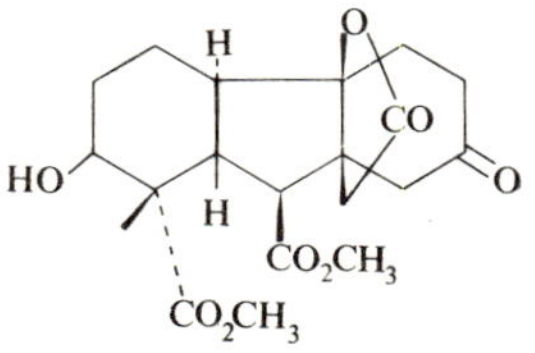

LVII

Moreover, the glycol (LII) as an allylic alcohol, was oxidized with manganese dioxide to an $\alpha\beta$-unsaturated ketone (λ_{max} 240 ϵ 17,000) carrying two substituents on the double bond. This established the presence of the grouping ($-\overset{\text{OH}}{\overset{|}{\text{C}}}\text{H}-\overset{\text{OH}}{\overset{|}{\text{C}}}\text{H}-\text{CH}{=}\text{C}\langle$) in the dicarboxylic acid (LII). On heating at 90° or under reflux in toluene and subsequent methylation the product yielded a neutral monomethyl ester (LI) isomeric with methyl gibberellate. This rearrangement occurs under mild basic conditions possibly by a concerted cyclic mechanism. When the reaction was carried out in D_2O and there was no incorporation of deuterium at position 10a—evidence which was used to suggest that this centre retained the more stable β-configuration.

Unlike the 7α-gibbane keto-ester (LIV) which underwent epimerization at position 4b in boiling 3N hydrochloric acid, the keto-ester (LV) was largely stable. However, treatment of the keto-ester (LV) with 6N hydrochloric acid [42] gave an equilibrium mixture of the starting material, the gibb-4a(4b)-ene (LVI) and a γ-lactone assigned the structure (LVII). It was the optical rotatory dispersion curve of this ketone which shed doubt on the original α-assignment to the 4b proton. Its 7-deoxy relative was obtained[42,51] by Clemmensen reduction of the keto-acid related to (62). The relactonization of various gibb-4a(4b)-enes has been studied.[45,46,66]

In an interesting acylation reaction with zinc and acetic anhydride,

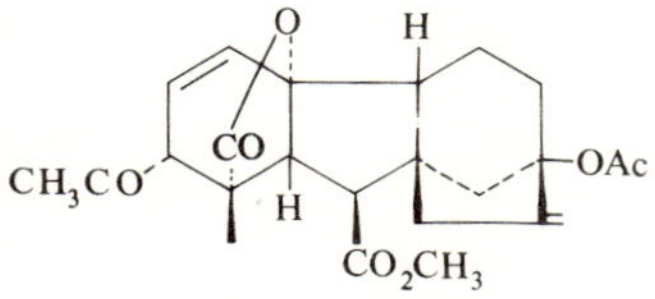

LVIII

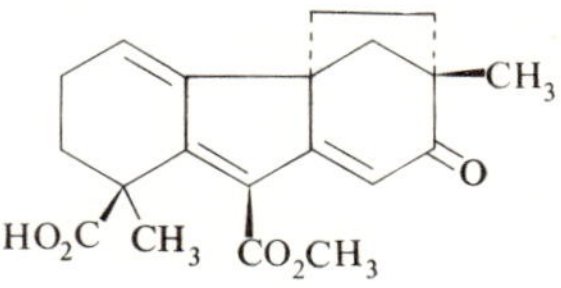

LIX

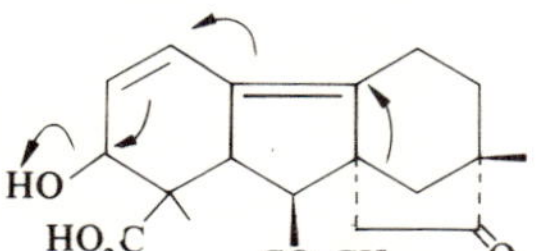

LX

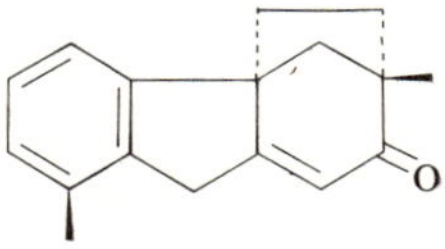

LXI

methyl gibberellate and its 2-*O*-acetyl derivatives give a 2-acetyl compound (LVIII).[67] Gibberellic acid in cold concentrated sulphuric acid gives an intense wine-red colour with a strong blue fluorescence which forms the basis of its fluorometric estimation.[12,25,68] A compound which can be reversibly converted into the fluorogen in sulphuric acid has been isolated and shown[68] to have the trienone structure (LIX) arising from a series of Wagner–Meerwein rearrangements (LX). Its structure rests upon mild dehydrogenation to an aromatic $\alpha\beta$-unsaturated ketone (LXI) and on more vigorous dehydrogenation. Treatment of the 7α-gibbane alcohols obtained by reduction of (LIV) with phosphorus pentachloride led to a reversal of the Wagner–Meerwein rearrangement to give the 7-deoxygibberellin system. Reduction of a 7-tosylate with Raney nickel also gave a route to the 7-deoxygibberellins. The bridgehead 7-tosylate undergoes a remarkable methanolysis to form a 7-methyl ether.[97]

3.9. *The C-20 Gibberellins*

A dicarboxylic acid, $C_{20}H_{28}O_4$, gibberellin A_{12} (LXII), was isolated[70] from *Gibberella fujikuroi* in low yield. The nuclear magnetic resonance spectrum revealed a gibbane skeleton which was confirmed[70,71] by partial synthesis from 7-hydroxykaurenolide. On treatment with alkali the 7-epitoluene-*p*-sulphonate (LXIII) of 7-hydroxykaurenolide gave a low

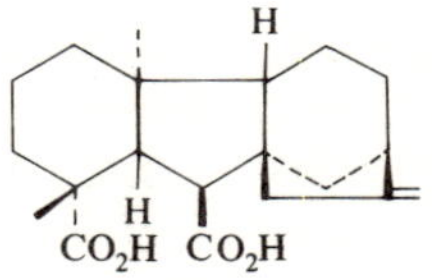

LXII

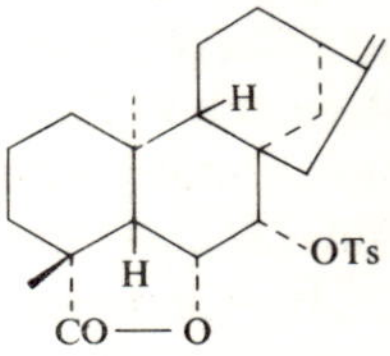

LXIII

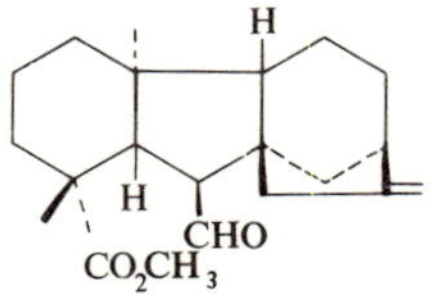

LXIV

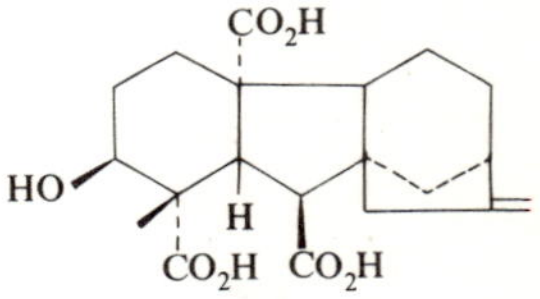

LXV

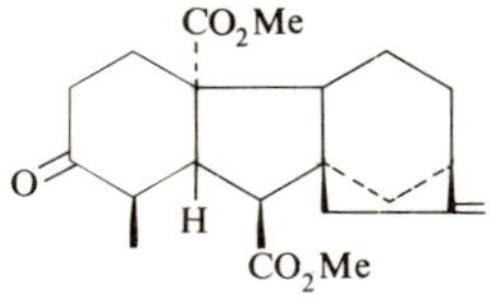

LXVI

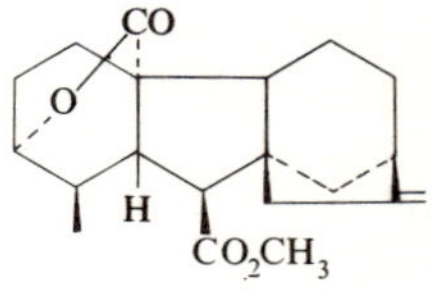

LXVII

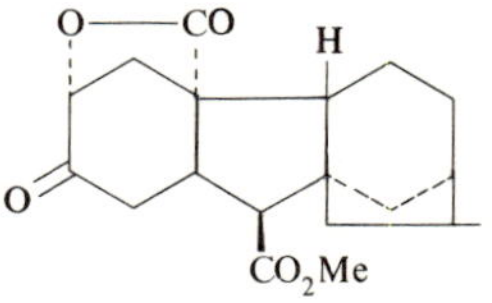

LXVIII

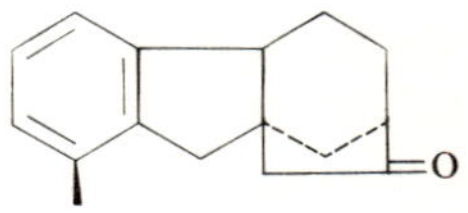

LXIX

yield of an aldehyde (LXIV) which was oxidized to the corresponding gibbane acid, the dimethyl ester of which was identical to that of gibberellin A_{12}. The monohydroxytricarboxylic acid, gibberellin A_{13} (LXV), isolated[72] from a mutant of *Gibberella fujikuroi* and from the 917 strain to which the enzyme inhibitor MER-29 (Triparanol) had been added. The nuclear magnetic resonance spectrum of its monoacetoxytrimethyl ester revealed five pendant groups and this together with the presence of the characteristic 10:10a quarter suggested a gibbane skeleton. Two of the carboxyl groups (at C-1 and 4a) were readily related through anhydride formation. One of these carboxyl groups was shown to be β- to the secondary hydroxyl group since on oxidation of the latter to a ketone it was lost as carbon dioxide. Furthermore, the n.m.r. spectrum of the dimethyl ester of this norketone (LXVI) showed, in contrast to its parent, a secondary methyl group. The infrared spectrum of the norketone showed it to be a cyclohexanone. Reduction of the ketone readily gave a δ-lactone (LXVII) involving the 4a carboxyl from which the structure of ring A of gibberellin A_{13} was deduced. The optical rotatory dispersion curve of the 2-ketone enabled the absolute stereochemistry to be assigned as in

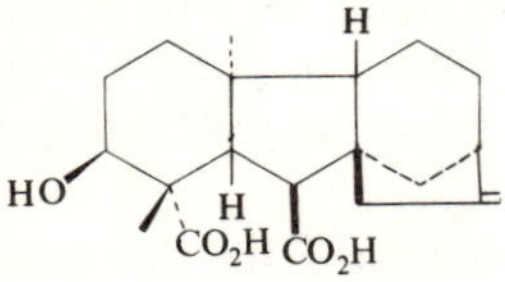

LXX

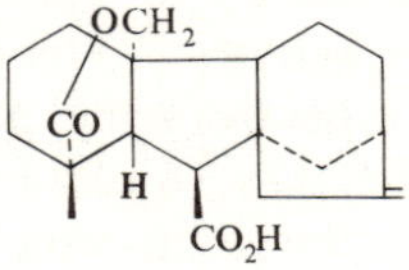

LXXI

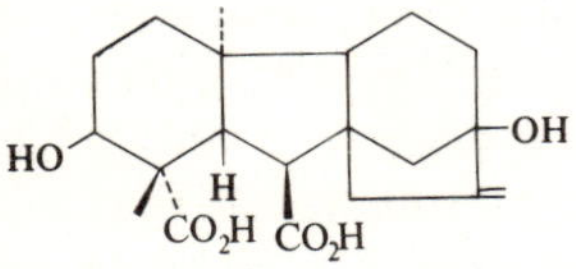

LXXII

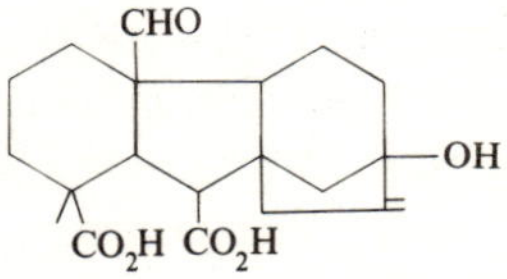

LXXIII

(LXV). Bromination of the ketone and dehydrobromination with collidine gave a γ-lactone (LXVIII) again establishing the presence of an angular 4a carboxyl. Ozonolysis of the double bond gave formaldehyde and cyclopentanone characteristic of the terminal methylene grouping of the gibberellins. Dehydrogenation of this norketone gave a gibbane derivative (LXIX) also isolated by dehydrogenation of gibberellin A_9. In confirmation of the proposed stereochemistry particularly at C-4b, (–)-19-hydroxykaurene was incorporated by the mould into gibberellin A_{13}.

Gibberellin A_{14} has been[73] shown to possess the structure (LXX). A δ-lactone gibberellin A_{15}, isolated[74] from the mould has spectral properties consistent with the formulation (LXX). Recently two C-20 gibberellins, (LXXII) A_{18} and (LXXIII) A_{19}, have been isolated[75,76] from

Lupinus luteus and bamboo shoots. The 2-hydroxy derivative of gibberellin A_{19} (A_{23}) has also been isolated from *Lupinus luteus* whilst gibberellin A_{17} has been identified[98] as the tricarboxylic acid corresponding to gibberellin A_{19}.

3.10. *Gibberellins in Higher Plants*

The search for these gibberellins has been facilitated by the development of a number of sensitive thin layer chromatographic methods.[77,78] In addition a number of sensitive bioassay methods are available using *inter alia* pea seedlings,[5] dwarf maize mutants[79] and cucumber hypocotyls.[80]

The occurrence of microgram amounts of gibberellins in higher plants has been established in a number of cases. Gibberellic acid and gibberellins A_1, A_4, and A_7 have been identified in an acidic extract of the seed of *Echinocystis macrocarpa*.[81] Gibberellic acid has also been identified in immature barley[82] and grass seed, Zea mays[76] and along with gibberellins A_1, A_5, A_6 and A_8 in *Phaseolus coccineus*[83] and *multiflorus*.[52–55] Gibberellin A_1 has been isolated from *P. vulgaris*,[84] and from *Citrus unshui*.[85] In addition crude extracts of many plants have been shown to have gibberellin-like activity.[86] The application of gas chromatography combined with mass spectrometry promises to be of considerable value in the identification of these gibberellins.[99]

Owing to the widespread effect of the gibberellins on the growth of higher plants, their biosynthesis has been the subject of several studies. Both acetate and mevalonate have been shown to be incorporated into gibberellic acid.[87] (−)-Kaurene,[88,89] (−)-kaur-16-en-19-ol and gibberellin A_{12}[90] have been shown to act as precursors of gibberellic acid demonstrating that ring contraction and oxygen particularly at C-2 and C-7, and the loss of the angular group, take place after the formation of the tetracyclic skeleton. The detail and significance of these results will be described in the chapter on biosynthesis. Although at the time of writing there is no complete total synthesis of the gibberellins a number of very closely related compounds have been synthesized. These results will be described in the chapter on synthesis.

REFERENCES

1. T. Yabuta and Y. Sumiki, *J. Agric. Chem. Soc.* (Japan), **14**, 1526 (1938).
2. T. Yabuta and T. Hayashi, *J. Agric. Chem. Soc.* (Japan), **15**, 257 (1939).
3. P. J. Curtis and B. E. Cross, *Chem. and Ind.*, 1066 (1954).
4. J. F. Grove, *Quart. Rev.*, **15**, 56 (1961).
5. P. W. Brian, J. F. Grove, and J. MacMillan, *Prog. Chem. Org. Nat. Prod.*, **18**, 350 (1960).
6. Cf. F. H. Stodola, *Source Book on Gibberellin*, 1828–1957, U.S. Dept. of Agriculture (1958).
7. G. M. Simpson, *Bibliography of the Gibberellins*, Univ. of Saskatchewan (1963).

8. R. KNAPP (Ed.), *Eigenschaften und Wirkungen der Gibberelline*, Springer-Verlag (1961).
9. *Régulateurs Naturels de la Croissance Végétale*, Centre Natl. Recherche Sci., Paris, (1964).
10. P. W. BRIAN, *Biol. Rev. Cambridge Phil. Soc.*, **34**, 37 (1959).
11. L. G. PALEG, *Ann. Rev. Plant Physiol.*, **16**, 291 (1965).
12. B. E. CROSS, *J. Chem. Soc.*, 4670 (1954).
13. T. YABUTA, Y. SUMIKI, K. ASO, T. TAMURA, H. IGARASHI and K. TAMARI, *J. Agric. Chem. Soc.* (Japan), **17**, 730, 894, 975 (1941).
14. P. W. BRIAN, J. F. GROVE, H. G. HEMMING, T. P. C. MULHOLLAND, and M. RADLEY, *Plant. Physiol.*, **33**, 329 (1958).
15. T. P. C. MULHOLLAND and G. WARD, *J. Chem. Soc.*, 4676 (1954).
16. B. E. CROSS, J. F. GROVE, J. MACMILLAN and T. P. C. MULHOLLAND, *Chem. and Ind.*, 954 (1956).
17. B. E. CROSS, J. F. GROVE, J. MACMILLAN and T. P. C. MULHOLLAND, *J. Chem. Soc.*, 2520 (1958).
18. T. YATAZAWA and Y. SUMIKI, *J. Agric. Chem. Soc.* (Japan), **25**, 503 (1952).
19. A. MORISON and T. P. C. MULHOLLAND, *J. Chem. Soc.*, 2536 (1958).
20. T. P. C. MULHOLLAND, *J. Chem. Soc.*, 2693 (1958).
21. A. J. BIRCH, R. W. RICKARDS, H. SMITH, J. WINTER and W. B. TURNER, *Chem. and Ind.*, 401 (1960).
22. J. F. GROVE and T. P. C. MULHOLLAND, *J. Chem. Soc.*, 3007 (1960).
23. J. S. MOFFATT, *J. Chem. Soc.*, 3045 (1960).
24. K. GERZON, H. L. BIRD, and D. O. WOOLF, *Experientia*, **13**, 487 (1957).
25. K. KAVANAGH and N. R. KUZEL, *J. Agric. Food Chem.*, **6**, 459 (1958).
26. B. E. CROSS, R. N. SPEAKE and J. R. HANSON, *J. Chem. Soc.*, 3555 (1965).
27. J. F. GROVE, J. MACMILLAN, T. P. C. MULHOLLAND, and W. B. TURNER, *J. Chem. Soc.*, 3049 (1960).
28. P. M. BOURN and W. KLYNE, *J. Chem. Soc.*, 2044 (1960).
29. P. M. BOURN, J. F. GROVE, T. P. C. MULHOLLAND, B. K. TIDD, and W. KLYNE, *J. Chem. Soc.*, 154 (1963).
30. B. E. CROSS, J. F. GROVE, J. MACMILLAN, T. P. C. MULHOLLAND and N. SHEPPARD, *Proc. Chem. Soc.*, 221 (1958).
31. B. E. CROSS, J. F. GROVE, J. MACMILLAN, J. S. MOFFATT, T. P. C. MULHOLLAND, J. C. SEATON, and N. SHEPPARD, *Proc. Chem. Soc.*, 302 (1959).
32. B. E. CROSS, *J. Chem. Soc.*, 3022 (1960).
33. B. E. CROSS and P. H. MELVIN, *J. Chem. Soc.*, 3038 (1960).
34. N. SHEPPARD, *J. Chem. Soc.*, 3040 (1960).
35. J. R. HANSON, *J. Chem. Soc.*, 5036 (1965).
36. B. E. CROSS, J. F. GROVE, P. MCCLOSKEY, T. P. C. MULHOLLAND, and W. KLYNE, *Chem. and Ind.*, 1345 (1959).
37. G. STORK and M. NEWMAN, *J. Amer. Chem. Soc.*, **81**, 5518 (1959).
38. O. E. EDWARDS, A. NICOLSON, J. W. APSIMON, and W. B. WHALLEY, *Chem. and Ind.*, 624 (1960).
39. D. C. ALDRIDGE, J. F. GROVE, R. N. SPEAKE, B. K. TIDD, and W. KLYNE, *J. Chem. Soc.*, 143 (1963).
40. B. E. CROSS, J. F. GROVE and A. MORRISON, *J. Chem. Soc.*, 2498 (1961).
41. S. MASAMUNE, *J. Amer. Chem. Soc.*, **83**, 1515 (1961).
42. D. C. ALDRIDGE and J. F. GROVE, *J. Chem. Soc.*, 2590 (1963).
43. F. MCCAPRA, A. I. SCOTT, G. SIM, and D. W. YOUNG, *Proc. Chem. Soc.*, 185 (1962).
44. A. I. SCOTT, F. MCCAPRA, F. COMER, S. A. SUTHERLAND, D. W. YOUNG, G. A. SIM, and A. FERGUSON, *Tetrahedron*, **20**, 1339 (1964).
45. D. C. ALDRIDGE, J. F. GROVE, P. MCCLOSKEY and W. KLYNE, *J. Chem. Soc.*, 2569 (1963).
46. T. P. C. MULHOLLAND, *J. Chem. Soc.*, 2606 (1963).
47. J. F. GROVE, P. W. JEFFS, and T. P. C. MULHOLLAND, *J. Chem. Soc.*, 1236 (1958).
48. D. F. JONES, and P. MCCLOSKEY, *J. Appl. Chem.*, **13**, 324 (1963).

49. Y. Seta, N. Takahashi, H. Kitamura and Y. Sumiki, *Bull. Agric. Chem. Soc.* (Japan), **22**, 62, 429, 432 (1958).
50. H. Kitamura, Y. Seta, N. Takahashi, A. Kawarada and Y. Sumiki, *Bull. Agric. Chem. Soc.* (Japan), **23**, 498, 412, 493 (1959).
51. Y. Seta, N. Takahashi, H. Kitamura, M. Takai, S. Tamura, and Y. Sumiki, *Bull. Agr. Chem. Soc.* (Japan), **23**, 499 (1959).
52. J. MacMillan and P. J. Suter, *Naturwiss.*, **45**, 46 (1958).
53. J. MacMillan, J. C. Seaton and P. J. Suter, *Proc. Chem. Soc.*, 325 (1959).
54. J. MacMillan, J. C. Seaton and P. J. Suter, *Tetrahedron*, **11**, 60 (1960).
55. J. MacMillan, J. C. Seaton and P. J. Suter, *Tetrahedron*, **18**, 349 (1962).
56. B. E. Cross, R. H. B. Galt, and J. R. Hanson, *Tetrahedron Letters*, **15**, 18 (1960).
57. N. Takahashi, Y. Seta, H. Kitamura, and Y. Sumiki, *Bull. Agr. Chem. Soc.* (Japan), **21**, 396 (1957); **23**, 405 (1959).
58. B. E. Cross, R. H. B. Galt, and J. R. Hanson, *Tetrahedron*, **18**, 451 (1962).
59. D. C. Aldridge, J. R. Hanson and T. P. C. Mulholland, *J. Chem. Soc.*, 3539 (1965).
60. H. Kitamura, Y. Seta, N. Takahashi, A. Kawarada, and Y. Sumiki, *Bull. Agr. Chem. Soc.* (Japan), **21**, 71 (1957); **22**, 434 (1958); **23**, 408 (1959).
61. H. Kitamura, N. Takahashi, Y. Seta, A. Kawarada, and Y. Sumiki, *Bull. Agr. Chem. Soc.* (Japan), **23**, 344 (1959).
62. J. F. Grove, *J. Chem. Soc.*, 3545 (1961).
63. B. E. Cross, R. H. B. Galt, and J. R. Hanson, *Tetrahedron Letters*, **23**, 22 (1960).
64. J. R. Hanson and T. P. C. Mulholland, *J. Chem. Soc.*, 3550 (1965).
65. J. R. Hanson, *Tetrahedron*, **22**, 701 (1966).
66. K. Mori, M. Matsui, and Y. Sumiki, *Agr. Biol. Chem.* (Japan), **27**, 530 (1963); **28**, 179 (1964).
67. D. F. Jones, J. F. Grove, and J. MacMillan, *J. Chem. Soc.*, 1835 (1964).
68. R. N. Speake, *J. Chem. Soc.*, 7 (1963).
69. B. E. Cross, J. R. Hanson, and R. N. Speake, *J. Chem. Soc.* 3555 (1965).
70. B. E. Cross and K. Norton, *J. Chem. Soc.*, 1570 (1965).
71. R. H. B. Galt and J. R. Hanson, *J. Chem. Soc.*, 1565 (1965).
72. R. H. B. Galt, *J. Chem. Soc.*, 3143 (1965).
73. B. E. Cross, *J. Chem. Soc.*, 501 (1966).
74. J. R. Hanson, *Tetrahedron*, in the press.
75. K. Koshimizu, H. Fukui, T. Kusaki, T. Mitsui and Y. Ogawa, *Tetrahedron Letters*, 2459 (1966).
76. S. Tamura, N. Takahashi, N. Murofushi, S. Iriuchijima, J. Kato, Y. Wada, E. Watanabe, and T. Aoyama, *Tetrahedron Letters*, 2465 (1966).
77. J. MacMillan and P. J. Suter, *Nature*, **197**, 790 (1963).
78. D. F. Jones, *Nature*, **202**, 1309 (1964).
79. B. O. Phinney and C. A. West, *Ann. Rev. Plant Physiol.*, **11**, 411 (1960).
80. P. W. Brian and H. G. Hemming, *Nature*, **189**, 74 (1961).
81. See G. W. Elson, D. F. Jones, J. MacMillan and P. J. Suter, *Phytochemistry*, **3**, 93 (1964).
82. D. F. Jones, J. MacMillan and M. Radley, *Phytochemistry*, **2**, 307 (1963).
83. G. Sembdner, G. Schneider, J. Weiland and K. Schreiber, *Experientia*, **20**, 89 (1964).
84. C. A. West and B. O. Phinney, *J. Amer. Chem. Soc.*, **81**, 2424 (1959).
85. A. Karawada and Y. Sumiki, *Bull. Agr. Chem. Soc.* (Japan), **23**, 343 (1959).
86. J. Kato, W. K. Purves and B. O. Phinney, *Nature*, **196**, 687 (1962).
87. A. J. Birch, R. W. Rickards and H. Smith, *Proc. Chem. Soc.*, 192 (1959); *Tetrahedron*, **7**, 241 (1959).
88. B. E. Cross, R. H. B. Galt and J. R. Hanson, *J. Chem. Soc.*, 295 (1964).
89. J. E. Graebe, D. T. Dennis, C. U. Upper, C. A. West, *J. Biol. Chem.*, **240**, 1847 (1965).
90. B. E. Cross and K. Norton, *Chem. Comm.*, 535 (1965).

91. R. H. B. GALT, *Tetrahedron*, **24**, 1337 (1968).
92. N. TAKAHASHI, N. MUROFUSHI, T. YOKOTA, and S. TAMURA, *Tetrahedron Letters*, 1065 (1967).
93. N. TAKAHASHI, N. MUROFUSHI, T. YOKOTA, S. TAMURA, J. KATO and Y. SHIOTANI, *Tetrahedron Letters*, 4861 (1967).
94. K. SCHREIBER, G. SCHNEIDER and G. SEMBDNER, *Tetrahedron*, **22**, 1437 (1967); N. N. GIROTRA and N. L. WENDLER, *Tetrahedron Letters*, 6431 (1966).
95. J. MACMILLAN and R. J. PRYCE, *J. Chem. Soc* (*C*), 740 (1967).
96. I. A. GURVICH, I. M. MILSTEIN and V. F. KUCHEROV, *Tetrahedron Letters*, 4293 (1967).
97. J. MACMILLAN and R. J. PRYCE, *J. Chem. Soc.* (*C*), 550 (1967).
98. R. J. PRYCE and J. MACMILLAN, *Tetrahedron Letters*, 4173 (1967).
99. J. MACMILLAN, R. J. PRYCE, G. EGLINTON and A. MCCORMICK, *Tetrahedron Letters*, 2241, 5009 (1967); N. TAKAHASHI, N. MUROFUSHI, S. TAMURA, N. WASADA, H. HOSHINO, T. TSUCHIYA, T. AOYAMA, and H. MORITA, *Tetrahedron Letters*, 895 (1967).
100. J. MACMILLAN and N. TAKAHASHI, *Nature*, **217**, 170 (1968).

CHAPTER 4

THE STACHENE CLASS

THE stachene group of tetracyclic diterpenes represent an alternative mode of collapse of the carbonium ion arising from cyclization of pimaradiene.

4.1. *Hibaene*

The parent hydrocarbon of this group—hibaene—has been isolated in both enantiomeric forms from a number of sources. The enantiomer, m.p. 29·5–30° $[\alpha]_D - 49{\cdot}9°$ with the normal A/B fusion and thus related to (+)-kaurane, has been isolated[1] from *Thujopsis dolabrata*. The other enantiomer, stachene, has been isolated[2,3] from *Erythroxylon monogynum*. The hydrocarbon cupressene, isolated[4] from a number of Cupressus species, is identical to stachene.

The evidence for the structure of hibaene (I) rests upon degradation and a series of interrelationships with other compounds in this series. Thus the n.m.r. spectrum of hibaene itself showed four tertiary *C*-methyl resonances at τ 9·03, 9·15, 9·19 and 9·27 together with a *cis* disubstituted olefin (τ 4·39 and 4·64; J = 6·0 c/s). The presence of the latter was confirmed by hydrogenation and epoxydation. The epoxide of stachene occurs[5] naturally in *Erythroxylon monogynum*. Cleavage of the double bond with potassium permanganate led to a dicarboxylic acid which formed a six-membered anhydride. The latter on dehydrogenation gave pimanthrene. Hence the double bond formed part of a five-membered ring bridging the perhydrophenanthrene backbone. The clearest evidence for the position of ring D and its stereochemistry comes from the identity of the dihydrostachene (derived from *Erythroxylon monogynum*) and isostevane and the enantiomeric relationship between dihydrohibaene (from *Thujopsis dolabrata*) and isostevane.[1] Furthermore, hydroboration of hibaene gave a C_{15} (II) and C_{16} ketone (III). The latter showed a rotatory dispersion curve of the same shape but opposite sign to that of isosteviol (IV) confirming the enantiomeric relationship of the form from *Thujopsis dolabrata*. Comparison[6] of the shielding effect of the C_{15}–C_{16} double bond on the angular C-10-methyl group with that of the C_8–C_{13} isomer, isohibaene (V) added further weight to this.

The partial synthesis[6] of isohibaene from isopimaradiene (VI) lay

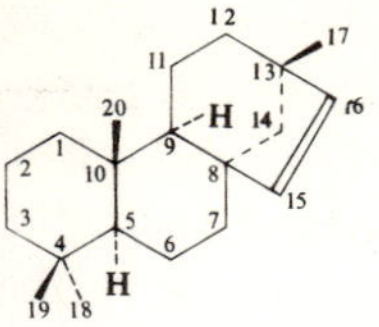

I 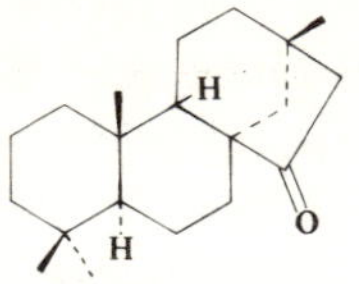 II 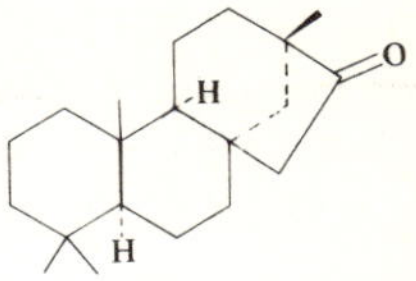 III

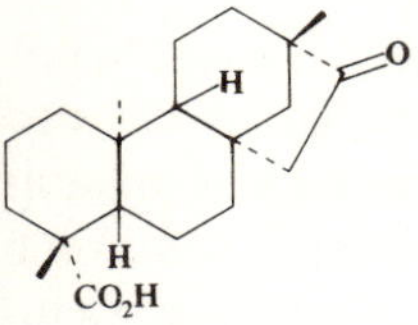

IV 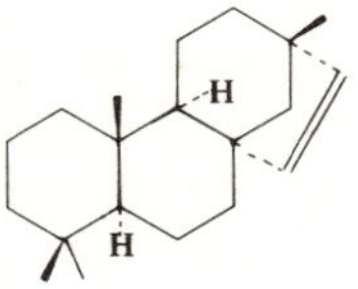 V 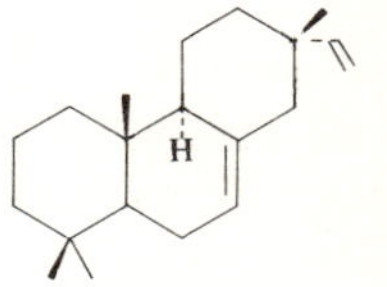 VI

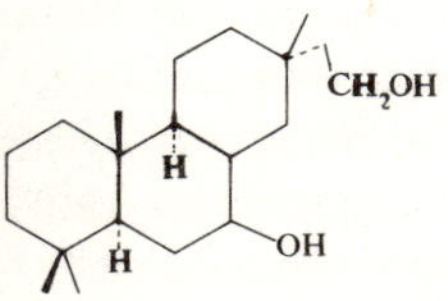

VII 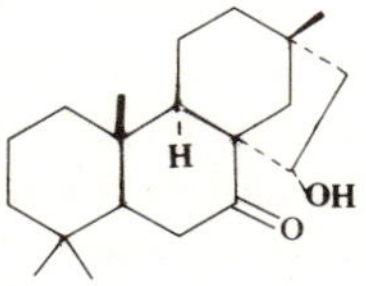 VIII

through hydroboration of the latter to a diol (VII) followed by oxidation to a keto-aldehyde and base-catalysed cyclization to a tetracyclic ketol (VIII). Dehydration and Wolff–Kishner reduction gave isohibaene (V).

The relationship between hibaene and (−)-kaurene was demonstrated[7] by treatment of the epoxide (IX) with boron trifluoride. A Wagner–Meerwein rearrangement to the unsaturated alcohol (X) ensued. Oxidation to a ketone and reduction of the latter to (−)-kaurene (XI) confirmed the structure of the product. The ease of this rearrangement is unusual in that it involves the conversion of a trans-*anti*-trans perhydrophenanthrene to a trans-*anti*-cis system.[8] This is described in Chapter 2.

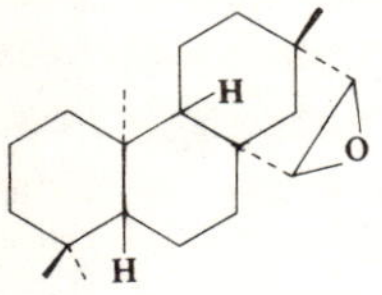

IX 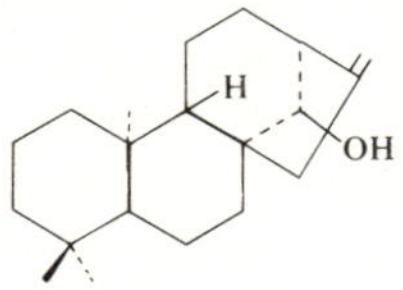 X 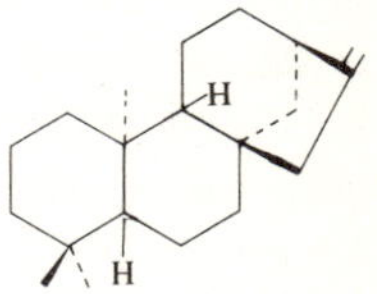 XI

4.2. *Stachenone*

A number of compounds of the stachene series have been isolated[9] from Tambooti wood (*Spirostachys africana*). This contains a ketone stachenone (XII), an α-ketol (XIII) and the corresponding diosphenol which were inter-related by oxidation. The presence of a disubstituted double bond in stachenone was demonstrated by cleavage of the corresponding α-glycol to a dicarboxylic acid. Dehydrogenation of this acid gave 1, 2, 7-trimethylphenanthrene in good yield compared with dehydrogenation of the parent diol and thus the double bond formed part of a bridge across a perhydrophenanthrene skeleton. Furthermore, the resistance to hydrolysis of the diester and the doublet character of the olefinic proton resonances suggested that the bridge was attached to a quaternary centre. These were in turn limited to 8 and 13. The position of the oxygen atoms was revealed by benzilic acid rearrangement of the diosphenol which led to the formation of an α-hydroxy-acid which was in turn cleaved to a norcyclopentanone. Thus the oxygen atom of stachenone was present in a six-membered ring. The isolation of 1, 2, 7-trimethylphenanthrene from dehydrogenation of the keto-acid (XIV) and of 1, 7-dimethylphenanthrene from stachenol defined its location at position 3. However, stachenol does not undergo the retropinacol rearrangement characteristic of a 4,4-dimethyl steroid. Optical rotatory dispersion measurements with the 3-ketone implied an antipodal A/B ring junction. The presence of a β-ring D bridge was considered[10] for stachenone. However, relationships with beyerol[11] and hence monogynol[2] and with isosteviol[6] together with a study of the n.m.r. spectra have now shown stachenone to have the structure and absolute stereochemistry (XII).

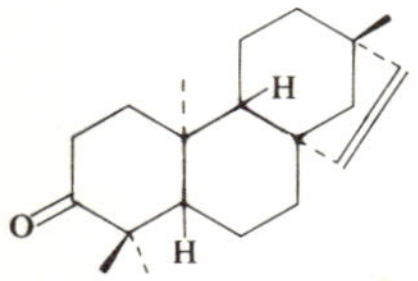

XII 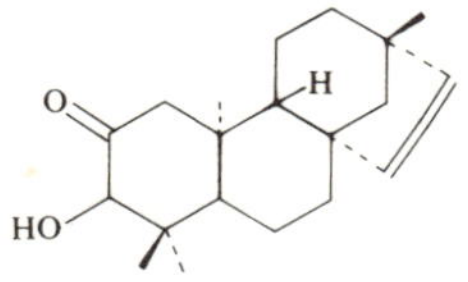 XIII 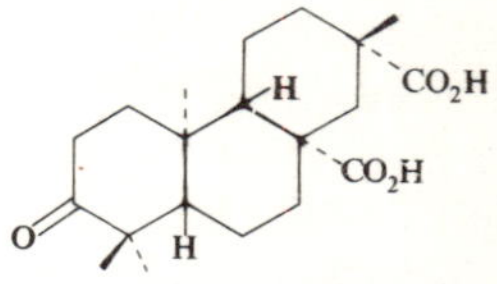 XIV

Examination of the n.m.r. spectrum of the α-ketol revealed the presence of three protons adjacent to the carbonyl group, one of which was also attached to a carbon atom bearing the hydroxyl of the ketol. Furthermore, reduction[12] of the ketol-tosylate led to 2-hydroxystachene which was oxidized to the corresponding 2-ketone, the latter containing four protons adjacent to the carbonyl group and hence the α-ketol was assigned the structure (XIII).

Treatment of the epoxide of stachenol acetate with boron trifluoride led to rearrangement[12] with the inversion of ring D and the formation of compounds with the kaurene skeleton.

4.3. *17-Hydroxystachene and Monogynol*

The Indian Devadaru wood *Erythroxylon monogynum* has been shown to contain a number of interesting tri- and tetracyclic diterpenes.[2,3,13] The tetracyclic constituents include the hydrocarbon, stachene, its corresponding epoxide, 17-hydroxystachene (XV), 19-hydroxystachene (monogynol) (XVI) together with 17, 19-dihydroxystachene.

The mono-ols were both converted to stachene. Thus monogynol was reduced through its 19-aldehyde and its derived ethylene thioketal, whilst the toluene-*p*-sulphonate of 17-hydroxystachene underwent hydrogenolysis with lithium aluminium hydride. Cleavage of the double bond of monogynol to a dicarboxylic acid followed by dehydrogenation gave pimanthrene. The stereochemistry of monogynol at position 4 as 19-hydroxystachene was apparent from the nuclear magnetic resonance spectra which showed an AB quartet (τ 6·53, 6·14, J = 11·5 c/s; acetate τ 6·08, 5·66 J = 11·0 c/s; aldehyde τ 0·27) typical of an axial hydroxymethyl group.[14] The pK^{MCS} of the related dihydro acid (8·59) belongs to the 19-position. Confirmation of this was received by a partial synthesis from the kaurenoid diterpene, steviol.

Steviol (XVII) has been related to (−)-kaurene and is of known stereochemistry (see section 2.3). On treatment with mineral acid steviol undergoes a Wagner-Meerwein rearrangement to form the keto-acid, isosteviol (IV) which has been shown to possess the stachene skeleton. Reduction of this keto-ester under catalytic conditions or with sodium borohydride leads to the 16α-alcohol. The toluene-*p*-sulphonate on treatment with collidine underwent elimination to form the Δ^{15}-olefin. Reduction of the ester with lithium aluminium hydride formed the required alcohol (XVI).

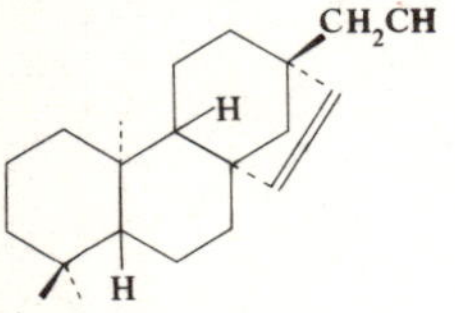

XV

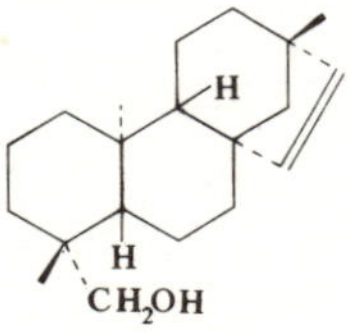

XVI

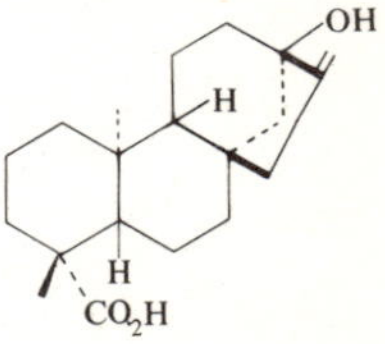

XVII

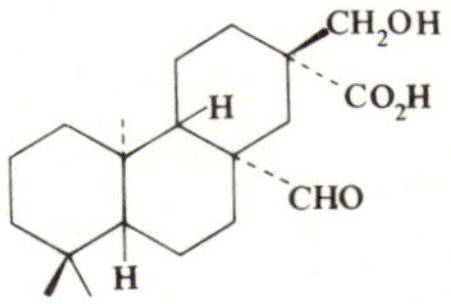

XVIII

The structure of 17-hydroxystachene followed from cleavage of the olefin with potassium permanganate and sodium periodate of the 17-acetate. Hydrolysis gave a hydroxy-aldehyde-acid (XVIII) isolated as its methyl ester. Oxidation of the latter gave a malonic half-ester which readily decarboxylated.[2]

4.4. *Beyerol*

The heartwood of *Beyeria leschenaultii* contains[16] a triol, beyerol (XIX), which occurs as its 17-monocinnamate. The presence of three reactive hydroxyl groups was demonstrated by the ready formation of triacyl derivatives. Oxidation of beyerol to a ketoaldehydic acid (XX) showed that these comprised one secondary and two primary alcohols. The presence of a 1:3 glycol, indicated by the formation of a chlorophosphochloridate and an ethylidene derivative, was confirmed by mild treatment of the ketoaldehydic acid with base to form a norketo-acid. The n.m.r. spectrum of the methyl ester of the latter contained resonances due to a secondary methyl group in contrast to the parent triol. The substitution pattern and position of oxygenation of this norketone was revealed by bromination and dehydrobromination of its dihydro derivative which led to an $\alpha\beta$-unsaturated ketone (λ_{max} 228 m$\mu\epsilon$ 11,000). This contained (from its n.m.r. spectrum) a *cis*-disubstituted double bond lacking allylic protons. Further bromination and dehydrobromination led to a trieneone (λ_{max}^{EtOH} 227 (ϵ 10,000), 258 (ϵ 5,600) and 309 (ϵ 6,600)) (XXI) analogous to a degradation product of cafestol (section 2.10). The n.m.r. spectrum of the trienone contained a vinylic methyl and two olefinic quartets neither showing allylic coupling. This clearly defined the position of the 1:3 glycol on ring A. Support for this came from the partial benzoylation of beyerol which gave a mono and a dibenzoate. Dehydration of the latter in which both primary groups were acylated, followed by hydrolysis gave anhydrobeyerol (XXII) containing a new *cis*-disubstituted olefin possessing two allylic protons.

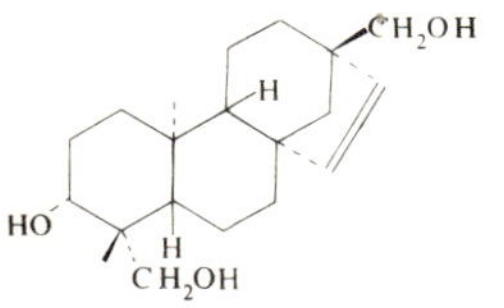

XIX 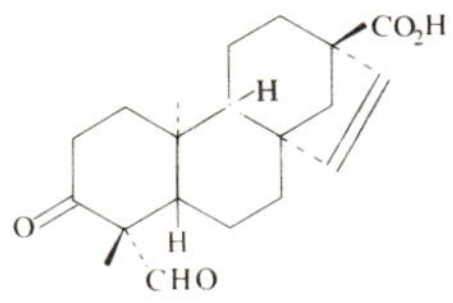 XX 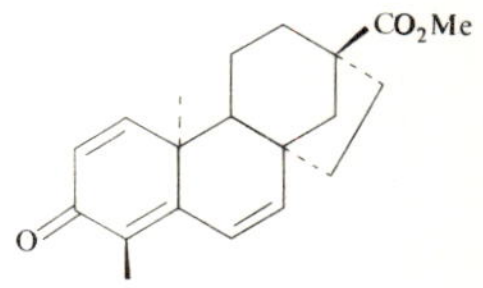 XXI

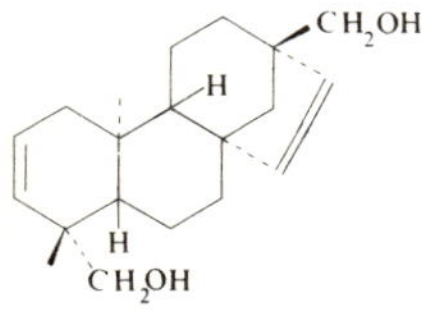

XXII 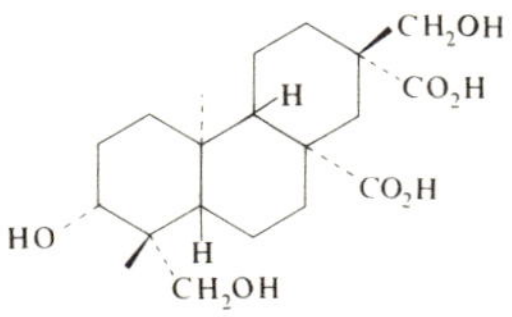 XXIII 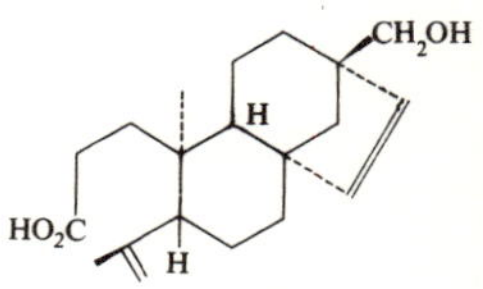 XXIV

The remote primary hydroxyl was attached to a quaternary centre since on oxidation it gave a tertiary carboxylic acid.

The ready hydrogenation, epoxide formation and osmylation to a pentanol revealed the presence of one double bond in beyerol. Cleavage of this olefin led to a dicarboxylic acid (XXIII) which reversibly formed a six-membered cyclic anhydride (ν_{max} 1800 and 1761 cm^{-1}). The latter was dehydrogenated to pimanthrene. Furthermore, the protons of this *cis*-disubstituted olefin showed no allylic coupling and hence the double bond was attached to fully substituted carbon atoms. The relationship of the 17-primary alcohol to this double bond was established by blocking the 1:3 glycol of the dicarboxylic acid (XXIII) as its ethylidene derivative and then oxidizing the remaining primary alcohol to a carboxylic acid. This readily decarboxylated. The stereochemistry of beyerol was assigned[11] on the following evidence. The optical rotatory dispersion curve of the 3-ketone indicated an antipodal A/B fusion. The position of the 19-aldehyde and acetoxymethyl proton resonances established their axial conformation and hence α-configuration. The shielding effect of the $\Delta^{15,16}$ double bond on the C-20 proton resonances showed[6,11] that these two functions were *cis* to one another. The α-configuration of the bridge was also demonstrated by comparison of the optical rotatory dispersion curves of the 15 and 16 ketones with the corresponding compounds derived from (+)-phyllocladene and (−)-kaurene. Hence beyerol was assigned the absolute stereochemistry (XIX). It was related to isostevane by reduction of the 17, 19-dibenzylthioether and to stachenol by reduction of the corresponding 3-hydroxy-17, 19-dibenzylthioether. 6β, 17-Dihydroxybeyer-15-en-3-one and its 6-acetate together with the 3, 4-secocarboxylic acid (XXIV) have been isolated[17] from a different variety of *Beyeria leschenaultii* 3α,17, 19-Trihydroxybeyer-15-ene and the three possible combinations of 3α,17 and 19-diols have been isolated[18] from *Helichrysum dendroideum.*

REFERENCES

1. Y. Kitahara and A. Yoshikoshi, *Tetrahedron Letters*, 884 (1964); *Bull. Chem. Soc.* (Japan), **37**, 890 (1964).
2. R. D. G. Murray and R. McCrindle, *Chem. and Ind.*, 500 (1964).
3. A. H. Kapadi and Sukh Dev, *Tetrahedron Letters*, 1171 (1964).
4. L. H. Briggs, R. C. Cambie, P. S. Rutledge and W. D. Stanton, *Tetrahedron Letters*, 2223 (1964).
5. A. H. Kapadi and Sukh Dev, *Tetrahedron Letters*, 2751 (1964).
6. E. Wenkert, P. W. Jeffs and J. R. Mahajan, *J. Amer. Chem. Soc.*, **86**, 2218 (1964).
7. A. H. Kapadi and Sukh Dev, *Tetrahedron Letters*, 1255 (1965).
8. R. P. Linstead, R. E. Whetstone and P. Levine, *J. Amer. Chem. Soc.*, **64**, 2014 (1926).
9. W. H. Baarschers, D. H. S. Horn and L. R. Johnson, *J. Chem. Soc.*, 4046 (1962).
10. A. I. Scott, F. McCapra, F. Somer, S. A. Sutherland, D. W. Young, G. A. Sim, and G. Ferguson, *Tetrahedron*, **20**, 1339 (1964).
11. P. R. Jefferies, R. S. Rosich and D. E. White, *Tetrahedron Letters*, 1793 (1963).
12. J. R. Hanson, *Tetrahedron*, **23**, 793 (1967).
13. R. C. Gupta and M. S. Muthana, *J. Ind. Inst. Sci.*, **36A**, 76,122 (1954).
14. A. Gaudemer, J. Polonsky and E. Wenkert, *Bull. Soc. Chim.*, 407 (1964).
15. J. R. Hanson, *Chem. and Ind.*, 1579 (1964).
16. P. R. Jefferies, R. S. Rosich, D. E. White and M. C. Woods, *Aust. J. Chem.*, **15**, 521 (1962).
17. E. L. Ghisalberti and P. R. Jefferies, *Tetrahedron Letters*, 6323 (1966); *Aust. J. Chem.*, **21**, 439 (1968).
18. H. A. Lloyd and H. M. Fales, *Tetrahedron Letters*, 4891 (1967).

CHAPTER 5

THE TETRACYCLIC DITERPENE ALKALOIDS

THE borderline between terpene and alkaloid metabolism shows an interesting overlap amongst the diterpene alkaloids. In contrast to the normal alkaloid biosynthesis from simple amino-acids, the nitrogen atom may be introduced at a much later stage in biosynthesis. The C_{20}–C_{22} alkaloids form a closely related group divided by the presence of bicyclo-3,2,1- and bicyclo-3,2,2-octane systems for rings C and D, into two classes – the garrya alkaloids and the atisine alkaloids. Derived from these is a group of more complex hexa- and heptacyclic bases with a rearranged C-19-carbon skeleton, described in Chapter 6. The chemistry of these alkaloids has been reviewed.[-5]

5.1. *The Garrya Alkaloids*

Alkaloids were originally detected in *Garrya fremontii* and *Garrya racemosa* in 1877 but it was not until 1946 that garryine (I) and veatchine (II) were isolated[6] from *G. veatchii*. Garryfoline, veatchine and cuauchichicine (III) have been isolated[7] subsequently from *G. laurifolia*. Cuauchichic resin was used in Mexican folk medicine as a remedy for diarrhoea whilst the extract of the bark and leaves of *Garrya elliptica* gave a bitter decotion used as a febrifuge.

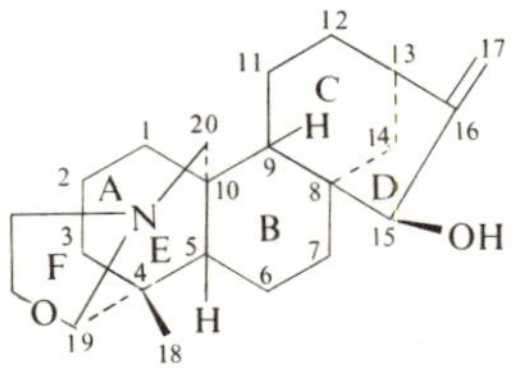

I

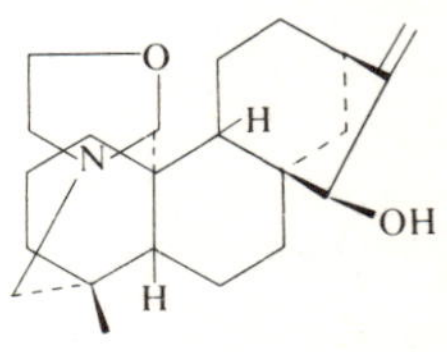

II

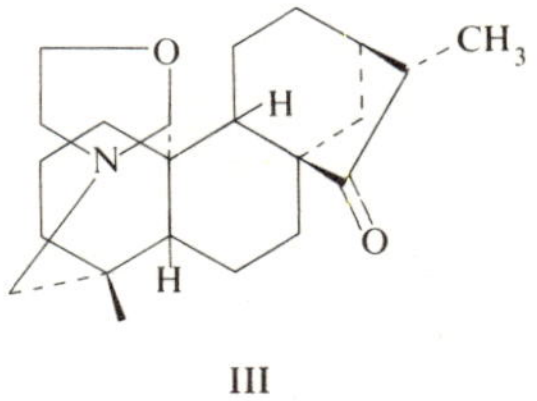

III

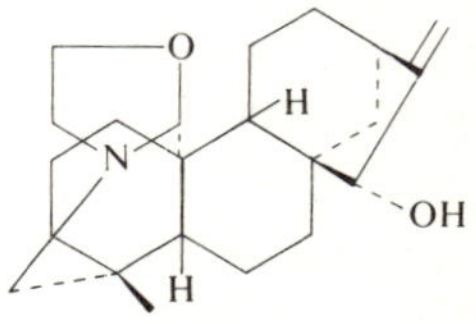

IV

Garryine, veatchine, garryfoline, and cuauchichicine are $C_{22}H_{33}O_2N$ isomers. Thus veatchine, which is a strong base, p*K* 11·5, is isomerized by alkali to the weaker base garryine (p*K* 8·5). Garryfoline (IV) which is a C-15 epimer of veatchine, was isomerized by acid to cuauchichicine.

5.2. *Garryine and Veatchine*

Garryine contained[8] one C-methyl, a hydroxyl, and a terminal methylene. Both garryine and veatchine gave dihydroveatchine (V) on reduction with lithium aluminium hydride and the same tetrahydroveatchine by catalytic hydrogenation of the terminal methylene group. Thus the alkaloids contained[9,10] isomeric carbinolamine ethers, owing their strong basicity to their ability to form anhydronium salts.

Dehydrogenation experiments revealed the nature of the carbon skeleton. Thus dehydrogenation of veatchine or garryine with selenium gave a good yield[11] of 1-ethyl-7-methylphenanthrene and an azaphenanthrene shown by X-ray analysis[12] and synthesis[13] to be 3-aza-7-ethyl-1-methylphenanthrene. Evidence for the position and substitution of additional carbocyclic ring came from a number of oxidative experiments.

Pyrolysis of either veatchine or garryine gave two isomeric azomethine bases. The non-ketonic material (VI) was reconverted[14] to garryine by reduction with lithium aluminium hydride to a secondary base (VII), alkylation with ethylene bromohydrin and reformation of the oxazolidine ring by an unusual oxidation with osmium tetroxide. The other ketonic product was a cyclopentanone (ν_{max} 1735 cm^{-1}) arising through allylic rearrangement. The presence of this allylic alcohol on ring D was substantiated by oxidation of the secondary base (VII) with chromium trioxide in pyridine to an $\alpha\beta$-unsaturated ketone (λ_{max} 236 mμ log ϵ 4·0). The points of fusion of this five-membered ring to the perhydrophenanthrene skeleton were shown by oxidation with potassium permanganate. Mild oxidation of garryine gave oxogarryine (ν_{max} 1618 cm^{-1}) formulated as (VIII) with a six-membered lactam. On the other hand, oxidation of veatchine gave two isomeric lactams, oxoveatchines A and B, formulated as (IX) (ν_{max} 1700 cm) and (X) (ν_{max} 1630 cm^{-1}). More vigorous oxidation of veatchine led to the cleavage of ring D and the formation of the dicarboxylic acids (XI) and (XII). Dehydrogenation of (XI) gave 1-methylphenanthra-7-yl carboxylic acid and pimanthrene. Reduction of the dimethyl ester followed by dehydrogenation gave pimanthrene. This evidence led to the proposed carbon skeleta.

Veatchine, the stronger base, was assigned the structure (II) since conversion of C_{20} to a trigonal centre in the azomethine base involved the greater release of compression energy and is thus the more facile process. Some further evidence came from dehydrogenation of methyldihydrogarryine obtained from garryine and methyl magnesium iodide. The azaphenanthrene obtained on dehydrogenation was 3-aza-1,2-dimethyl-7-ethylphenanthrene.

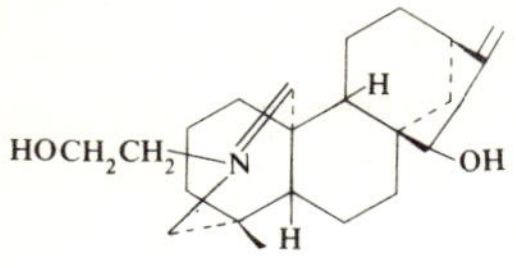

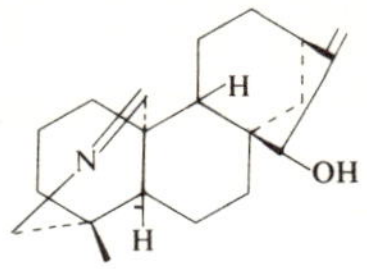

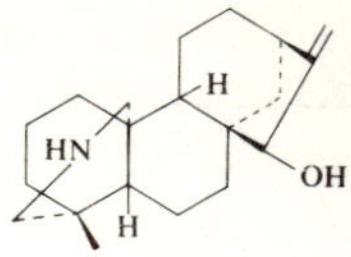

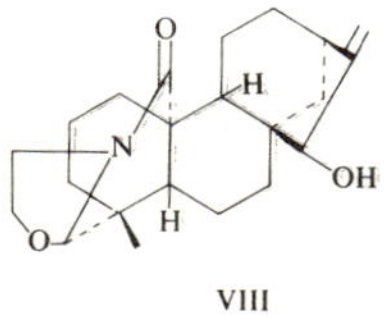

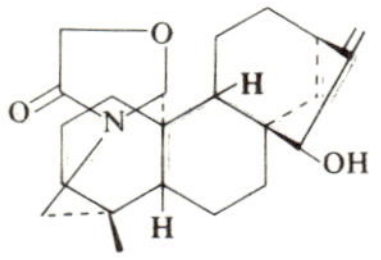

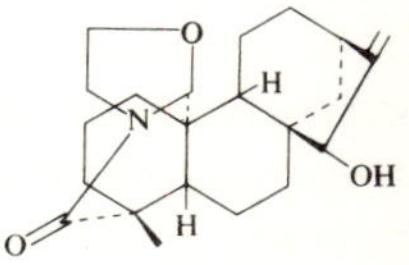

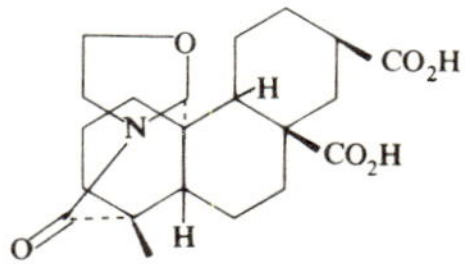

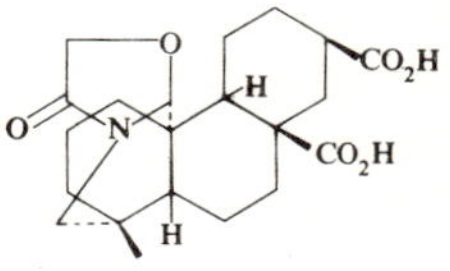

5.3. *Cuauchichicine and Garryfoline*

Two alkaloids, cuauchichicine (III) and garryfoline (IV) were isolated[7] from the bark of the Mexican tree, *Garrya laurifolia*. The ketonic alkaloid, cuauchichicine contained a cyclopentanone and on pyrolysis gave the ketonic azomethine base (XIII) which had been isolated in the degradation of veatchine. This established the nature of the carbon skeleton. Cuauchichicine was a strong base (p*K* 11·8) and was isomerized by alkali to a weaker base, isocuauchichicine (p*K* 8·6) from which the attachment of the oxazolidine ring at C-20 in cuauchichicine followed.

The second alkaloid garryfoline (IV) was readily isomerized by mineral acid to cuauchichicine. The oxazolidine ring was reduced with lithium aluminium hydride to F-dihydrogarryfoline (XIV); formulated as the C_{15} epimer of dihydroveatchine. This relationship was established by oxidation of veatchine to an $\alpha\beta$-unsaturated ketone and reduction of both the ketone and the oxazolidine ring with lithium aluminium hydride to form F-dihydrogarryfoline.

The configuration of the secondary hydroxyl group in the C-15 epimers veatchine and garryfoline was assigned on the basis of the ready isomerization of the latter to cuauchichicine. The mediation of a non-classical carbonium ion (XV) involving C-12, 13 and 16 was proposed[15] for this isomerization. Of the two C-15 isomeric alcohols only one (IV) has a proton readily eliminated for this ketonization to occur. This structure was assigned to garryfoline. Furthermore reduction of F-dihydrocuauchichicine with lithium in liquid ammonium gave the more stable 15-epitetrahydroveatchine.

The absolute stereochemistry of these alkaloids was determined by a series of degradations[16–18] and optical rotatory dispersion measurements. The orientation of ring D was determined by oxidation of the terminal methylene of F-dihydrogarryfoline diacetate to an α-ketol acetate. Reductive deacetoxylation with calcium in liquid ammonia gave a cyclopentanone. The optical rotatory dispersion curve of this ketone exhibited a positive Cotton effect, similar to that of phyllocladene. The position of the first extremum of the Cotton effect of the keto-acetate derived from veatchine occurred at 342 $m\mu$ as compared with 327·5 mμ for the ketol of the garryfoline series. This supported the previous assignment of the stereochemistry of the corresponding acetate.

An attempt to elucidate the stereochemistry at C-9 failed at the stage of opening ring D lactone. However, garryfoline was degraded[17,18] to the diterpene hydrocarbon, (—)-β-dihydrokaurene, a minor hydrogenation

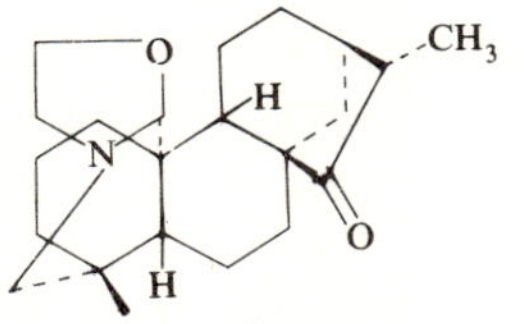

III

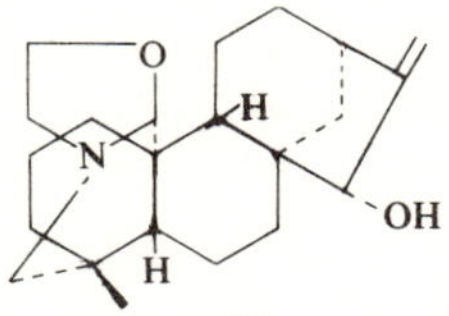

IV

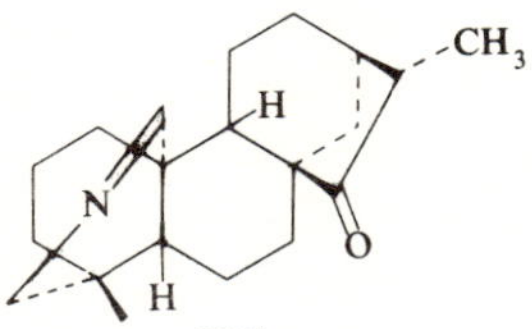

XIII

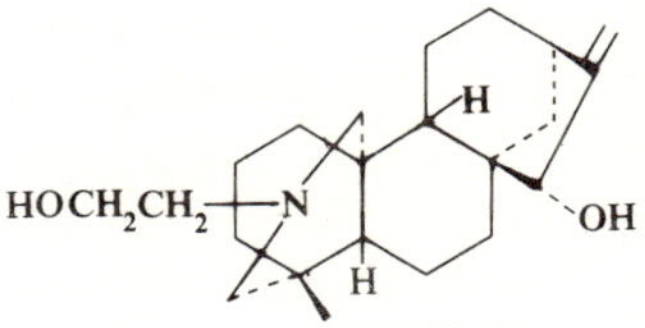

XIV

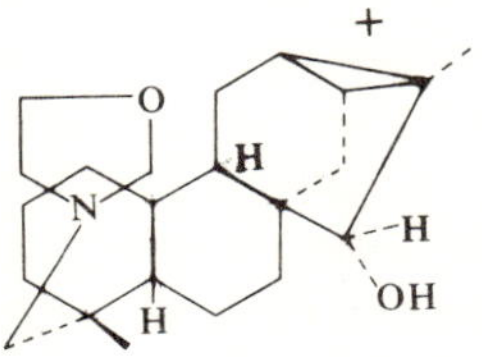

XV

product of (–)-kaurene. Elimination of the nitrogen ring was accomplished by treatment of the azomethine (XVI) with nitrous acid. Wolff–Kishner reduction of the resulting hemiacetal (XVII) effected simultaneous reduction of the 15-ketone and the masked 19-aldehyde to afford a C-20 primary alcohol (XVIII). The latter was oxidized to an aldehyde and again reduced by a vigorous Wolff–Kishner reduction to the diterpene hydrocarbon (XIX). The aldehyde and the corresponding acid behaved as very hindered groupings.

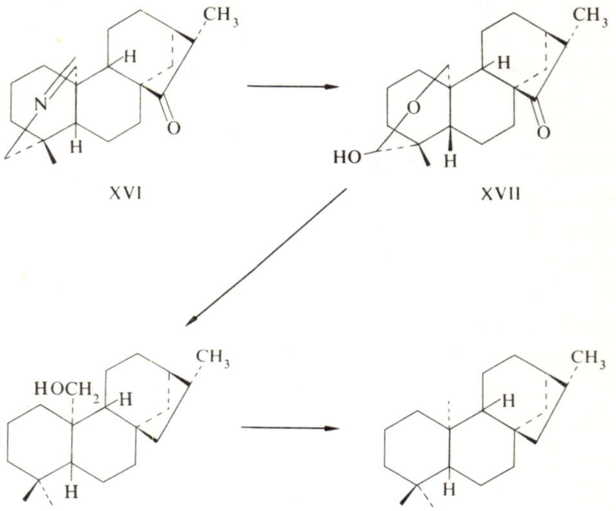

XVI XVII

XVIII XIX

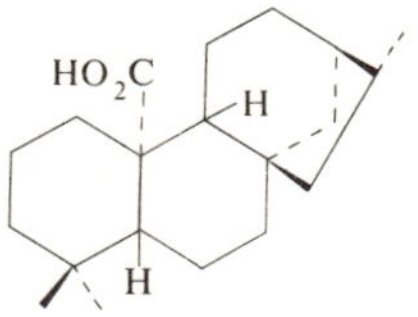

XX

The total synthesis of alkaloids of this series has been announced utilizing the carboxylic acid (XX) as an intermediate.

5.4. *Napelline and Songorine*

The alkaloid napelline (XXI) forms a link between the Garrya and atisine bases in that, although it was isolated[20] from *Aconitum napellus*, it possesses a kauranoid carbon skeleton. The initial investigations showed that it was a triol related to a naturally occurring keto-diol, napellonine (songorine) (XXII). The 15-monoacetate (XXIII) is the alkaloid, lucidusculine,[21–24] from *Aconitum lucidusculum.* Both napelline and songorine underwent the acid-catalysed rearrangement to ketonic derivatives characteristic of a kaur-16-en-15β-ol system. At one time napelline was formulated[25] as (XXIV). However, selenium dehydrogenation of songorine gave a trisubstituted phenanthrene which was eventually identified[26,27] as 1,9-dimethyl-7-ethylphenanthrene. This required a bond between C-20 and C-7, and precluded the formation of carbinolamine

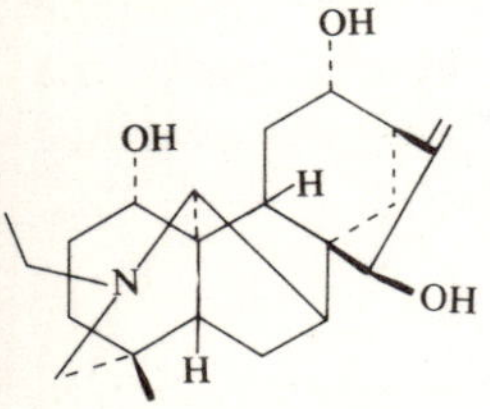
XXI

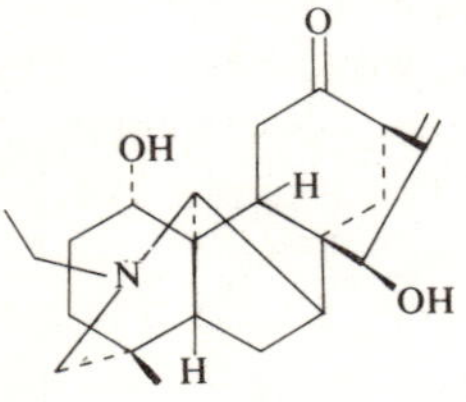
XXII

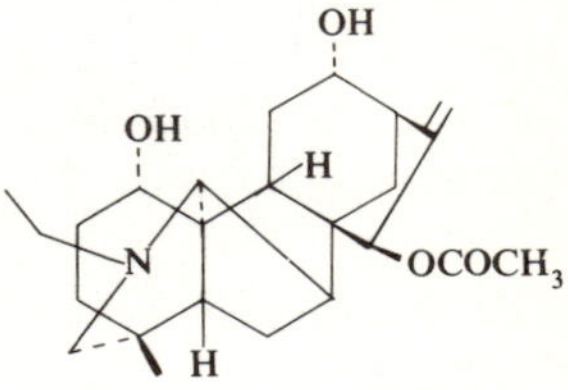
XXIII

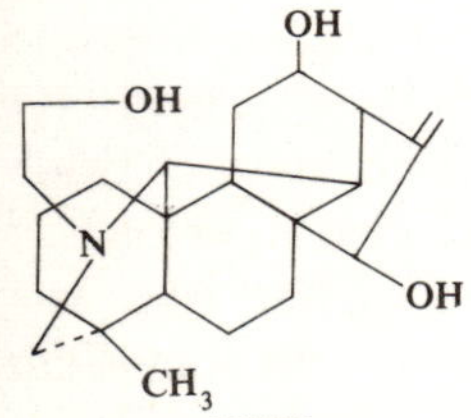
XXIV

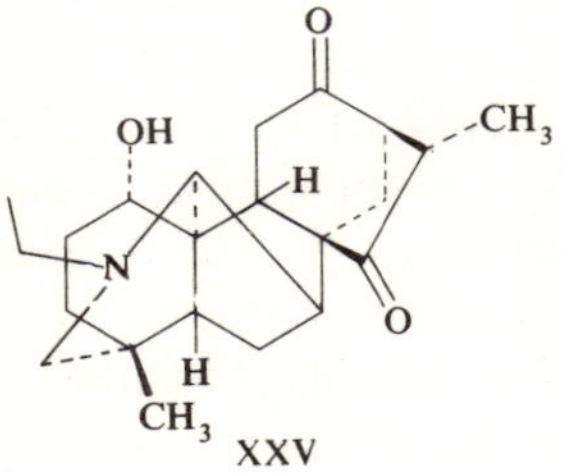
XXV

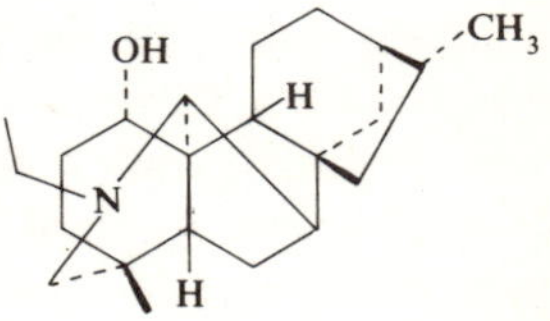
XXVI

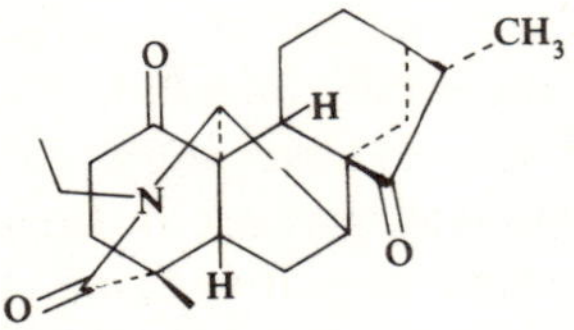
XXVII

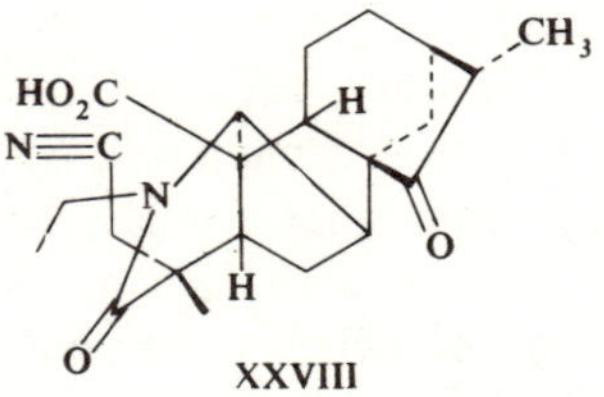
XXVIII

ethers involving C-20 which are then incompatible[28] with Bredt's rule. A re-investigation of the structure napelline indicated that it contained a N-ethyl group. However, dihydronapelline forms a carbinolamine ether by oxidation with silver oxide involving C-19 and the third hydroxyl group which was therefore located on ring A.

The location of this hydroxyl at C-1 arose as follows. Isosongorine (XXV), derived[29] from songorine by allylic rearrangement, on Wolff–Kishner reduction gave an alcohol, dideoxyisosongorine (XXVI) retaining the ring A hydroxyl. Oxidation of this alcohol gave a keto-lactam which incorporated 1·8 atoms of deuterium on equilibration with NaOD thus indicating the presence of methylene group adjacent to the keto function. The location of this ketone at C-1 followed from the conversion of the diketo-lactam (XXVII) to the ring A α-oximino ketone with isoamyl nitrite. Ring A was then cleaved by the rearrangement of this system with benzenesulphonyl chloride and alkali to the cyano-acid (XXVIII). The latter was stable to acid thus precluding the presence of a malonamide and hence a C-3 oxygen function. These transformations led to the proposal that songorine had the structure (XXII) whilst napelline was the corresponding ring C equatorial alcohol. X-ray analysis of the acetate, lucidusculine, confirmed this structure and provided evidence that it represented[23] the absolute configuration of songorine.

5.5. *Atisine Alkaloids*[4,5]

Atisine is the major alkaloid of the Indian medicinal plant *Aconitum heterophyllum*. Although it was described in 1877 and in subsequent years,[30] the correct molecular formula was not proposed[31] until 1937.

Atisine, $C_{22}H_{33}NO_2$ (XXIX) is a strong base (pK 12·2) which was isomerized to a weaker base iso-atisine[37] (XXX). Functional group analysis indicated the presence of an exocyclic methylene, a hydroxyl group and a C-methyl. The formation of diacetylatisine hydrochloride was originally taken as evidence for the presence of two hydroxyls.[32] However, location of the second oxygen in an oxazolidine ring was provided[33] by two lines of evidence. Oxidation of atisine with potassium permanganate gave[34,35] γ- and δ-lactam dicarboxylic acids (e.g. XXXI) the methyl esters of which showed no hydroxyl absorption in the infra-red[36] and no active hydrogen. Secondly, mild oxidation of atisine with chromium trioxide in pyridine led[33] to the formation of an $\alpha\beta$-unsaturated ketone (λ_{max} 236 mμ) indicative of an allylic alcohol. This atisone possessed no active hydrogen and no hydroxyl absorption in the infrared and hence the remaining oxygen atom was present in an ether ring. Reduction of atisine with hydride formed dihydro-atisine, lead tetra-acetate oxidation of which gave glyoxal, suggestive of a β-hydroxyethyl group.[38] Final confirmation of the presence of an oxazolidine ring came from its reconstitution.[38] Pyrolysis of atisine or better Hofmann elimination of diacetyl atisine hydrochloride led to an azomethine base (XXXII). Reduction of this with sodium borohydride and alkylation of the resulting secondary amine with ethylene chlorohydrin gave dihydroatisine. Oxidative cyclization of the β-hydroxyethyl group with osmium tetroxide gave isoatisine. A lactam lacking the β-hydroxyethyl side chain of dihydro-atisine formed[39] a minor product of the Sarett oxidation of atisine. Isoatisine on the other hand gave as a minor product the corresponding lactam retaining this side chain.

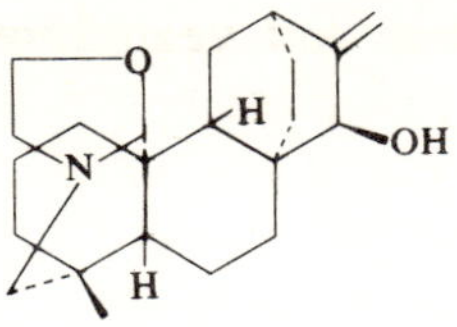

XXIX 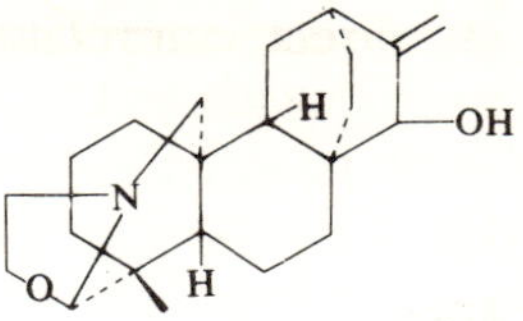 XXX

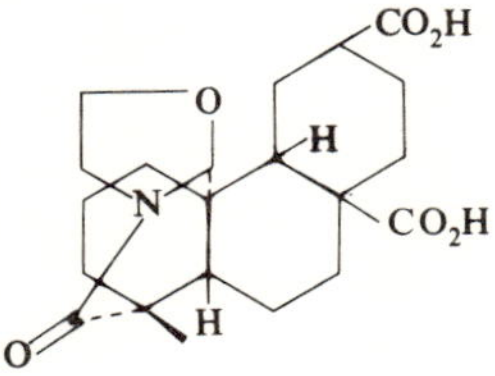

XXXI 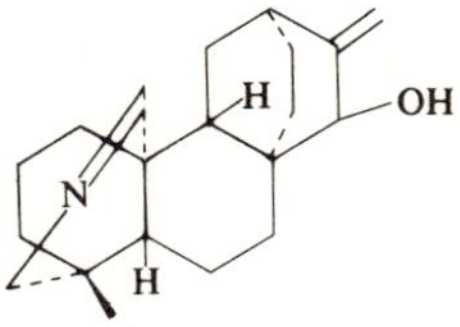 XXXII

Evidence bearing on the nature of the carbon skeleton came from dehydrogenation experiments which yielded 1-methylphenanthrene,[40] 1-methyl-6-ethylphenanthrene[41] and 3-aza-1-methyl-6-ethylphenanthrene.[42] Two pieces of evidence were used to establish the points of fusion of the fourth carbon ring and clarify the relative disposition of the hydroxy group and terminal methylene.

The azomethine (XXXII) on treatment with mineral acid gave a diol. The azomethine was then reduced and protected as the *N*-acetyl diol by acetylation and partial saponification.[43] Cleavage of this diol led to the 15:16-secoketo-acid which was in turn converted by Baeyer–Villiger oxidation to a bisnor-acetoxy-acid. Careful saponification gave the parent hydroxy-acid (more vigorous conditions led to lactonization) which was oxidized to a keto-acid. Dibromination and dehydrohalogenation of this gave a phenol (XXXIV) and a keto-γ-lactone (XXXV) thus demonstrating the relationship between the carboxyl group and the ketone in (XXXIII) and hence the size of ring D.[39] The enantiomer of this phenol was prepared[44] by photolysis of the azide of podocarpic acid methyl ether (XXXVI) to form a δ-lactam. Cleavage of the aromatic ether, reduction of the lactam to an aminophenol, acetylation and partial saponification completed the partial synthesis. This formed clear evidence for the antipodal nature of the A/B ring fusion. The second piece of evidence for the structure of ring D came from dehydrogenation experiments. The isolation of a number of 6-substituted phenanthrenes indicated that one terminus of ring D lay at that position. When the ring D oxygen function was removed 1-methyl-6-isopropylphenanthrene rather than 1-methyl-6-n-propyl phenanthrene was isolated[45] from dehydrogenation experiments. Had the alternative sequence of terminal methylene and hydroxyl group been present, a n-propyl would represent the residue of ring D.

A direct correlation of atisine and veatchine was achieved[46,47] via the bisnor-ester (XXXVII). Cleavage of ring D of the *N*-acetate derived from atisine utilizing the Rudloff–Lemieux procedure afforded the noracid (XXXVIII). Hunsdiecker degradation of the silver salt of the mono-methyl ester gave a poor yield of the bisnorbromoester from which bromine was reductively removed to form (XXXVII).

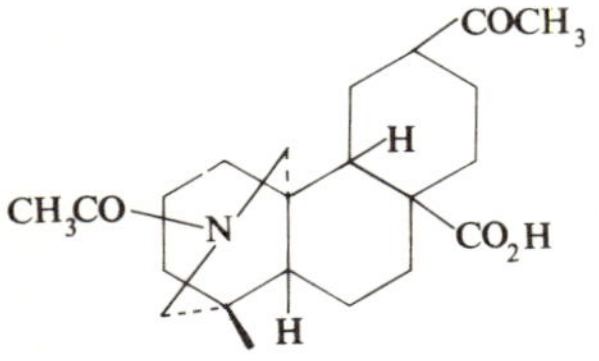

XXXIII 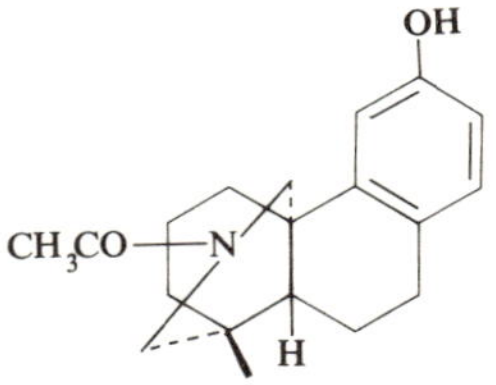 XXXIV 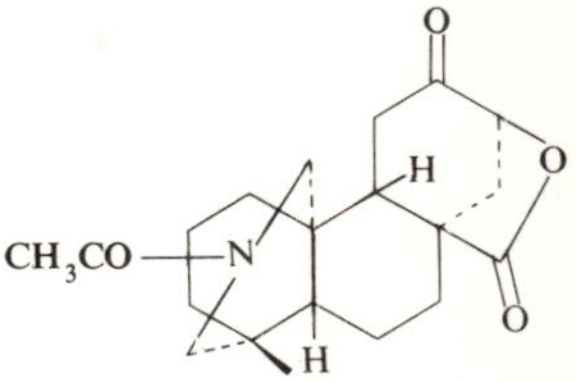 XXXV

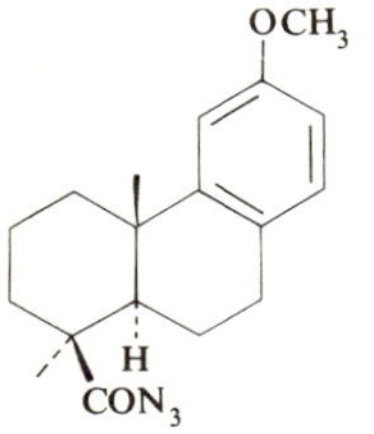

XXXVI 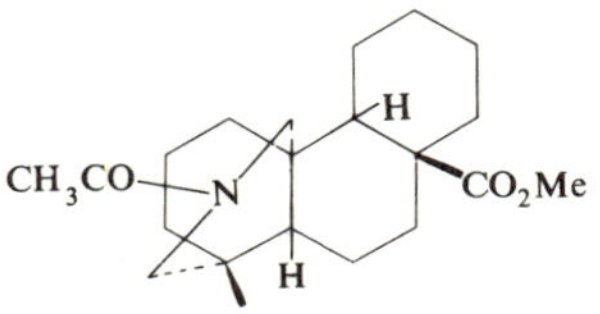 XXXVII 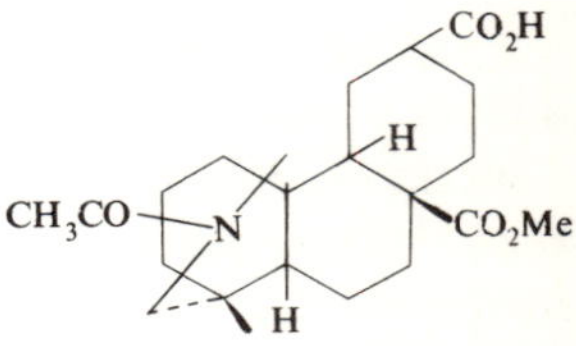 XXXVIII

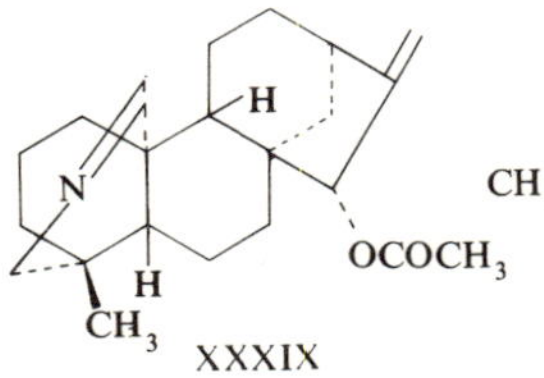

XXXIX 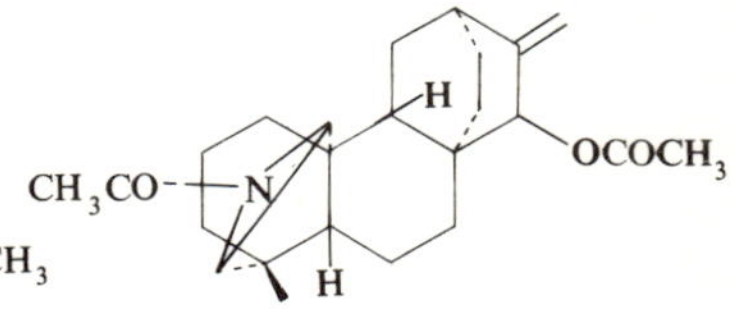 XL

Alternatively hydration of the azomethine (XXXII) gave a diol which on reduction, acetylation and partial saponification formed the *N*-acetyl diol. Cleavage of the diol led to the 15,16-secoketo-acid in turn converted by Baeyer–Villiger oxidation to a bisnoracetoxy-acid. Careful saponification gave the parent hydroxy-acid which was oxidized to the keto-acid. Reduction of the corresponding keto-ester through the ethylene thioketal then led to (XXXVII).

Veatchine was converted through the iminium diacetate chloride to the azomethine acetate (XXXIX) and thence by reduction acetylation, and partial saponification to an *N*-acetate. Cleavage of ring D by the Rudloff–Lemieux reagent gave a dicarboxylic acid. Partial saponification of the derived dimethyl ester gave a monocarboxylic acid the silver salt of which was subjected to the Hunsdiecker degradation. Reductive debromination then formed the required bisnor ester, identical to the product derived from atisine and thereby providing clear evidence for the common stereochemistry of the atisine and garrya alkaloids. Since the absolute stereochemistry of the latter was known, this clarified the absolute stereochemistry of the atisine series. This could be extended to a complete stereochemistry since there was evidence[43, 45] that indicated that the allyl alcohol occupied the *trans* bridge of the bicyclo-2,2,2-octane system relative to the heterocyclic ring.

A tentative assignment of the configuration of the secondary alcohol of atisine was made on the basis of the relative absorption of C-15 epimeric alcohols on alumina. The hydroxyl group and *N*-acetyl group were assumed to be on the same side of the molecule in the unnatural series since they were more strongly adsorbed.

The highly hindered environment of the oxazolidine ring leads to a number of unusual reactions particularly of its azomethine counterpart.[5] Thus the azomethine (XXXII) is remarkably resistant to the normal hydrolytic action of acids and bases.[48–50] The driving force for facile isomerization of atisine to isoatisine by base has been ascribed[5] to the interaction of the oxygen with C-11 and to the restriction which the oxazolidine ring places upon rotation of the C-10–C-20 bond in atisine preventing relief of the interactions with the ethylene bridge of ring D. The higher basicity of atisine is accounted for by the preponderance of the ternary iminium hydroxide[51, 52] of atisine in which C-20 is trigonal and the interactions of the tetragonal C-20 in the oxazolidine ring are relieved. These factors do not operate to the same extent in the iso bases. In the case of the salts those derived from the "normal" series have the less bulky trigonal carbon atom at C-20 and are therefore more stable than the "iso" salts. Thus refluxing isoatisinium chloride in dimethyl sulphoxide gives an 85 per cent yield of atisinium chloride. Since the normal salts are smoothly converted to the bases by mild treatment with alkali this provided a convenient means of reversing the "isobase" isomerization.

Reduction of the imino alcohol with zinc dust in acetic anhydride afforded as a major product the *O.N*-diacetate and a dimer as a byproduct. On the other hand prolonged refluxing of the imine with acetic anhydride led to the *N*-acetyl aziridine (XL). The synthesis of atisine and its relatives will be discussed in Chapter 7.

5.6. *Atidine and Ajaconine*

Atidine, $C_{22}H_{33}NO_3$ (XLI) was isolated[53] along with atisine from *Aconitum heterophyllum*. It was characterized as a keto-diol. Wolff–Kishner reduction of the keto-group led to dihydroatisine[54] thus establishing the carbon skeleton. Sodium borohydride reduction of the keto-group gave a mixture of epimers one of which was dihydroajaconine. Since atidine was unstable to alkali the presence of a β-hydroxyketone capable of undergoing retro aldol cleavage was suggested [cf. the synthesis of isohibaene]. This, taken with the evidence for the structure of ajaconine led to the structure (XLI) for atidine.

Ajaconine (XLII), an isomer of atidine, was first isolated[55,56] from *Delphinium ajacis* and characterized in 1945. Subsequently it was isolated from *D. consolida*. Ajaconine was related[57,58] to atisine by degradation to a common azomethine base (XLIII). Furthermore, the relationship to atidine and thence dihydroatisine clarified the position of the allylic alcohol system of ring D. Sodium borohydride reduction of the carbinolamine ether system, gave a dihydro base which formed a triacetyl derivative. This underwent the ready Hofmann-type elimination to give an azomethine base. This together with the high pK (11·3), and the formation of anhydronium salts led to the initial structure for ajaconine containing an atisine-like oxazolidine ring. However, subsequent work showed[59] that this involved the 7-oxygen atom. Evidence for the position of an oxygen atom at this centre came following the degradation. The diacetoxyazomethine obtained from Hofmann elimination was oxidized to a C_{19} acetoxynorketone. Wolff–Kishner reduction eliminated the oxygen functions on ring D and led to an azomethine mono-ol (XLIV). The corresponding ketone on bromination and dehydrobromination formed an $\alpha\beta$-unsaturated ketone with spectral properties consistent with a ring B ketone. In particular the ultraviolet spectrum (λ_{max} 250 mμ, calc. 244 mμ) showed an interaction with the nitrogen bridge.

Treatment of the methiodide of the azomethine mono-ol with strong base led to the formation of a carbinolamine ether (XLV). The rotation changes accompanying this reaction led to a reinterpretation of the structure originally assigned to ajaconine and its formulation as (XLII).

The juxtaposition of C-7 and C-20 functions led to an interesting internal hydride transfer reaction. The azomethine mono-ol was oxidized to the corresponding ketone and methylated. Treatment of the latter with strong base led to the iso compound (XLVI) and the hydroxy-lactam (XLVII).

5.7. *Ignavine and Hypoignavine*

Ignavine $C_{27}H_{31}NO_6$ was isolated[4] from *Aconitum sanyoense*,[60] *A. tasiromontanum*[60] and *A. japonicum*.[61] Saponification of ignavine liberated[60] benzoic acid and an anhydroignavinol, $C_{20}H_{25}NO_4$. On both saponification and acylation ignavine readily loses a mole of water in an ether formation reaction. Ignavine contains one double bond, shown[62,63] by ozonolysis to be the terminal methylene characteristic of the series.

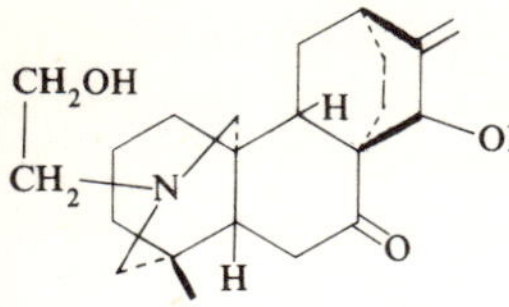

XLI 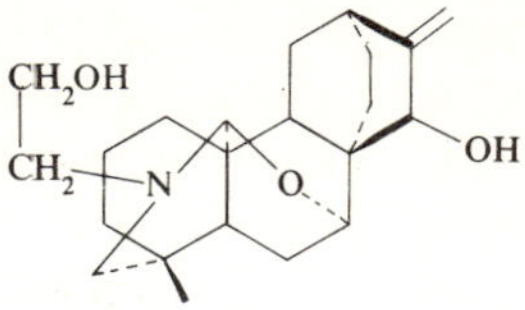 XLII 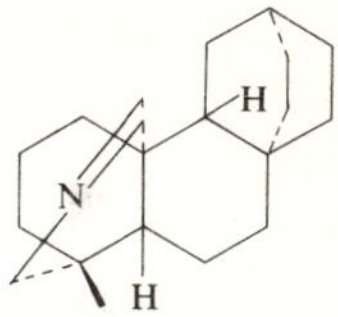 XLIII

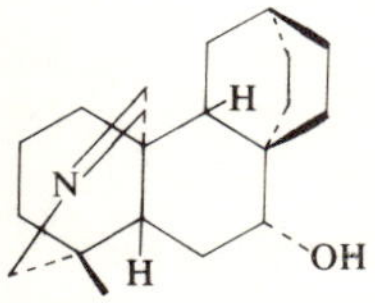

XLIV 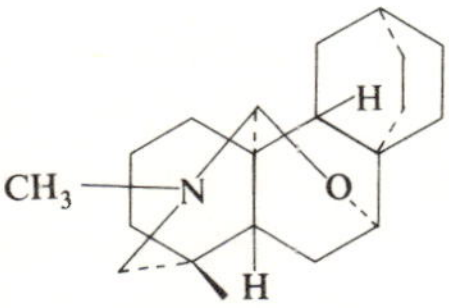 XLV 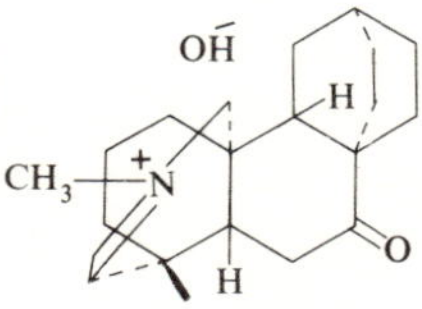 XLVI 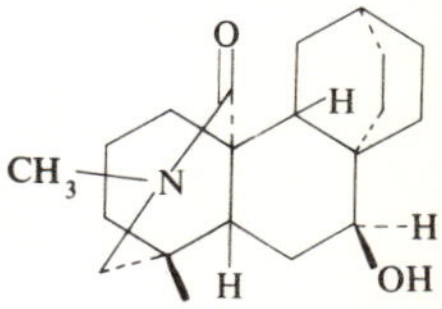 XLVII

Since the oxygen atoms are accounted for in hydroxyl groups the carbon skeleton must contain a further carbon–carbon bridge. The key to its position was provided by the characteristic selenium dehydrogenation pattern in which the phenanthrenes (XLVIII) to (L) were isolated.[64] Their structures were established by synthesis.[65]

Oxidation to an $\alpha\beta$-unsaturated ketone and allylic rearrangement revealed[63] the presence of the secondary allylic alcohol on ring D. The presence of an α-glycol system, partially masked as the benzoate in the parent alkaloid was established by periodate cleavage. The position of this on ring A was demonstrated by the oxidation of des-*N*-methylanhydroignavinol tribenzoate (derived from a Hofmann degradation of anhydroignavinol) to a lactam. Saponification and oxidative cleavage of the glycol gave a dicarboxylic acid which as a malonamide underwent ready decarboxylation. This led to the partial structure (LI) for anhydroignavinol.

Hypoignavine which occurs in *Aconitum sanyoense*,[66] is the benzoate of an alkamine hypoignavinol, $C_{20}H_{27}NO_4$. In many of its reactions[67] it parallels ignavine. It has been assigned the partial formula (LII) in which one hydroxyl group remains to be located.

5.8. *Kobusine and Pseudo-Kobusine*

Kobusine and pseudo-kobusine have been isolated from the roots of *Aconitum yesoensis*[68,69] and *A. sachalinense*.[70] Pseudo-kobusine [(LIII) or (LIV)] was shown to be a triol containing the typical allylic alcohol moiety of this group of alkaloids. Selenium dehydrogenation gave 1,7-dimethyl-6-n-propylphenanthrene indicative of the underlying carbon skeleton of the molecule and suggesting a close skeletal relationship to ignavine. The presence of a ketone masked as a $\rangle$N-$\overset{|}{\underset{|}{C}}$-OH group was

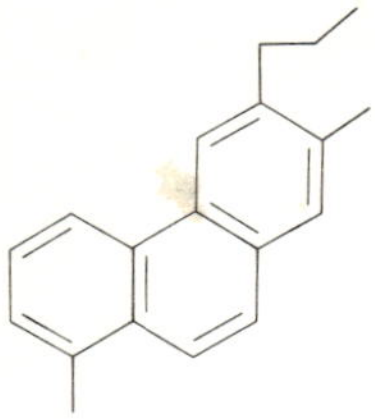

XLVIII 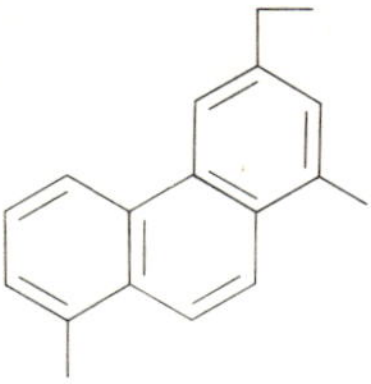 XLIX 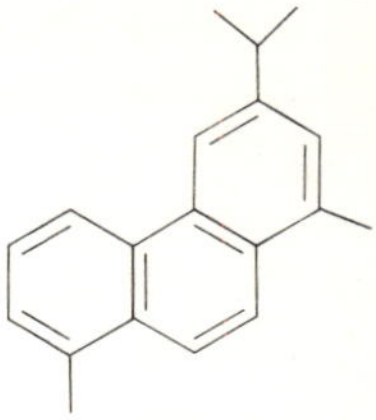 L

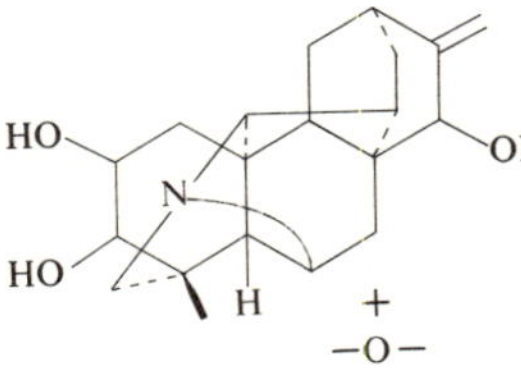

LI 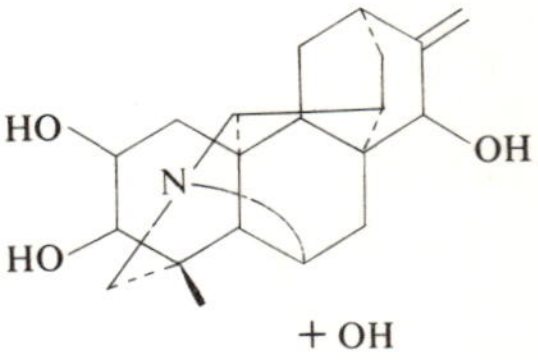 LII

revealed[71] by the reversible formation of an *N*-acetyl secopseudokobusine (LV), *N*-cyano derivative and *N*-methyl derivative. The influence of this tertiary hydroxyl on the methyl proton resonances in pseudokobusine defined the location of this group at C-6. The position of the third hydroxyl group was limited to two centres by oxidative cleavage of ring D. *N*-acetylsecopseudokobusine (LV) was oxidized with osmium tetroxide–sodium periodate to yield a monocarboxylic acid containing a hemiacetal. Oxidation of the monomethyl ester led to a γ-lactone (LVI) thus defining the location of the third hydroxyl with respect to the allylic alcohol.

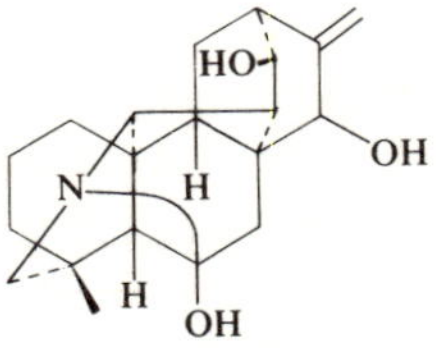

LIII 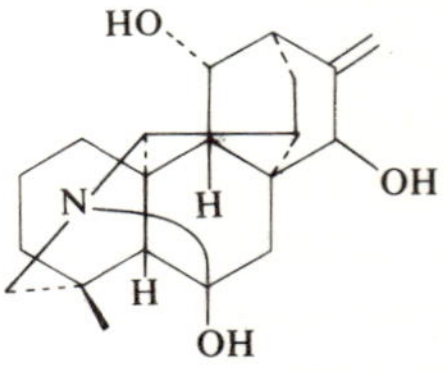 LIV

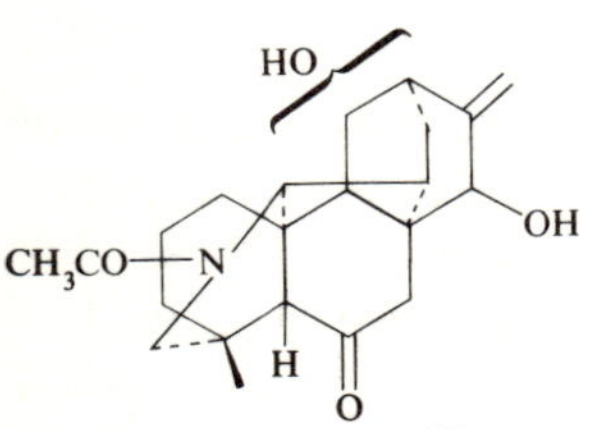

LV 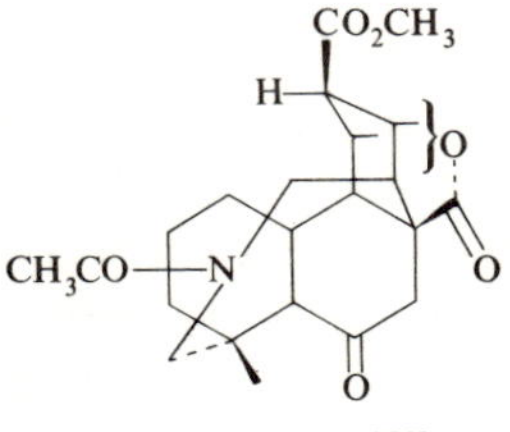 LVI 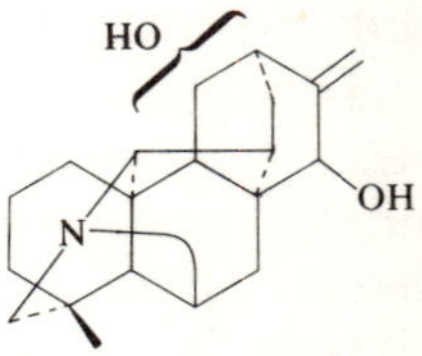 LVII

Pseudokobusine was related[72] to kobusine (LVII) by reductive removal of the tertiary hydroxyl group through its methane sulphonate.

Thus the two alkaloids possess the same carbon–nitrogen skeleton and the same two secondary hydroxyl groups.

5.9. *Hetisine*

Hetisine $C_{20}H_{27}O_3N$ (LVIII) co-occurs[73] with atisine in *Aconitum heterophyllum*. It is identical to delatine[74] from *Delphinium elatum*. It was characterized as a triol with a tertiary nitrogen atom lacking *N*-alkyl and methoxyl groups. The one double-bond was present as a terminal methylene. The alkaloid contained one *C*-methyl group. The solution of its structure was complicated by skeletal rearrangements and a number of proposals were rejected before X-ray analysis[75] clarified the problem.

Dehydrogenation gave a complex mixture from which pimanthrene was isolated. Other evidence for the nature of the skeleton came from the basicity (pK_a' 9·85) which was indicative of a quinuclidine structure.

Hofmann degradation was complicated by the intervention of a rearrangement. The first preparation of "hetisine" methiodide involved sufficiently vigorous conditions to bring about rearrangement to a carbon skeleton reminiscent of the hibaene series. The product (LIX) underwent a one-stage Hofmann degradation to give desmethylhetisine containing a *N*-methyl group, and new *C*-methyl group and only one double bond.

Desmethylhetisine (LX) did not contain carbonyl absorption and hence in the rearrangement (LVIII) to (LIX) the ketonic product must be masked by hemiketal formation. Hetisine gave mono and dicarbonyl derivatives; these were not conjugated with the terminal methylene.

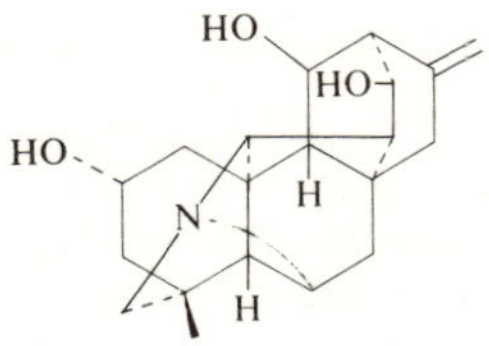

LVIII

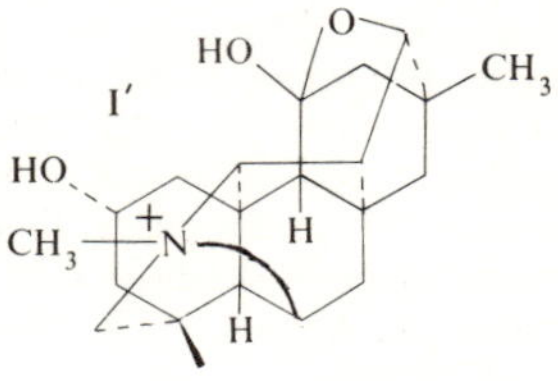

LIX

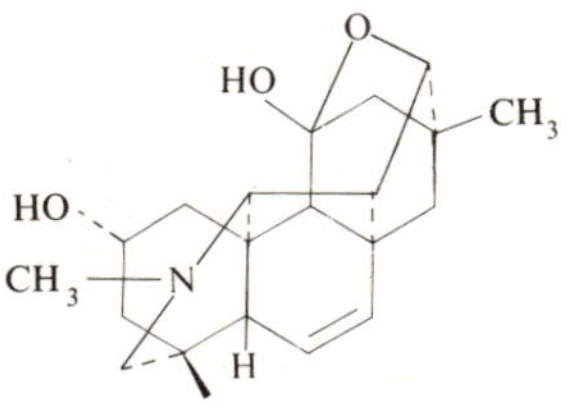

LX

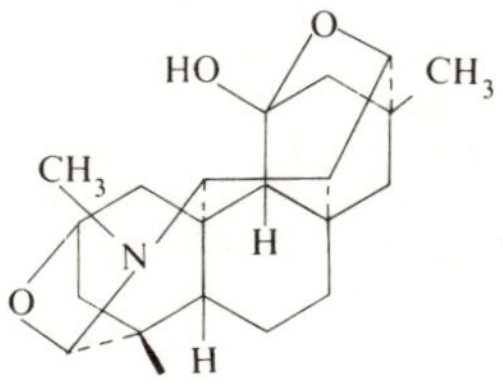

LXI

Dihydrohetisine undergoes Hofmann degradation without rearrangement. The structure of the oxidation product of hetisine with chromium trioxide in pyridine is at present obscure. However, oxidation of dihydrodesmethylhetisine with potassium permanganate leads to a carbinolamine ether (LXI) involving the ring A alcohol.

REFERENCES

1. K. WIESNER and Z. VALENTA, *Prog. Chem. Org. Nat. Prod.*, **16**, 26 (1958).
2. E. S. STERN, *The Alkaloids*, Ed. R. D. H. MANSKE, Vol. VII, p. 473, Academic Press, New York (1960).
3. A. R. PINDER, *Chemistry of Carbon Compounds*, Vol. IVC, Ed. RODD, ELSEVIER, (1962).
4. S. W. PELLETIER, *Tetrahedron*, **14**, 76 (1961).
5. S. W. PELLETIER, *Experientia*, **20**, 1 (1964); *Quart. Rev.*, **21** 525 (1967).
6. J. F. ONETO, *J. Amer. Pharm. Soc.*, **35**, 204 (1946).
7. C. DJERASSI, C. R. SMITH, A. E. LIPMANN, S. K. FIGDOR and J. HERRAN, *J. Amer. Chem. Soc.*, **76**, 5889; **77**, 4801 (1955).
8. K. WIESNER, S. K. FIGDOR, M. F. BARTLETT and D. R. HENDERSON, *Canad. J. Chem.*, **30**, 608 (1952).
9. K. WIESNER, R. ARMSTRONG, M. F. BARTLETT and J. A. EDWARDS, *J. Amer. Chem. Soc.*, **76**, 6068 (1954).
10. K. WIESNER and J. A. EDWARDS, *Experientia*, **11**, 255 (1955).
11. K. WIESNER, W. I. TAYLOR, S. K. FIGDOR, M. F. BARTLETT, R. ARMSTRONG and J. A. EDWARDS, *Chem. Ber.*, **86**, 800 (1953).
12. E. W. HUGHES and R. NATHAN, reported in ref. 13.
13. K. WIESNER, J. R. ARMSTRONG, M. F. BARTLETT and J. A. EDWARDS, *Chem. and Ind.*, **132**, 542 (1954).
14. M. F. BARTLETT, W. I. TAYLOR and K. WIESNER, *Chem. and Ind.*, 272 (1952); 173 (1953).
15. Cf. J. MACMILLAN and M. F. BARNES. *J. Chem. Soc.* (C), 361 (1967).
16. H. VORBRUGGEN and C. DJERASSI, *Tetrahedron Letters*, 119 (1961); *J. Amer. Chem. Soc.*, **84**, 2990 (1962).
17. E. MOSETTIG, P. QUITT, U. BERLINGER, J. A. WATERS, H. VORBRUGGEN and C. DJERASSI, *J. Amer. Chem. Soc.*, **83**, 3163 (1961).
18. C. DJERASSI, P. QUITT, E. MOSETTIG, R. C. CAMBIE, P. S. RUTLEDGE, and L. H. BRIGGS, *J. Amer. Chem. Soc.*, **83**, 3720 (1961).
19. S. MASAMUNE, *J. Amer. Chem. Soc.*, **86**, 288 (1964).
20. L. C. CRAIG and W. A. JACOBS, *J. Biol. Chem.*, **143**, 611 (1942).
21. H. SUGINOME and S. KAKIMOIO, *Bull. Chem. Soc.* (Japan), **32**, 352 (1959).
22. H. SUGINOME, T. AMIYA, and T. SHIMA, *Bull. Chem. Soc.* (Japan), **32**, 824, 113 (1959); **33**, 644, 1175 (1960).
23. A. SUZICKI, T. AMIYA, and T. MATSUMOTO, *Bull. Chem. Soc.* (Japan), **34**, 455, 898 (1961).
24. T. OKAMOTO, M. NATSUME, Y. IITAKA, A. YOSHINO and T. AMIYA, *Chem. and Pharm. Bull.*, **13**, 1270 (1965).
25. K. WIESNER, Z. VALENTA, J. F. KING, R. K. MAUDGAL, L. G. HUMBER, and S. ITO, *Chem. and Ind.*, 173 (1957).
26. A. D. KUZOVKOV, *J. Gen. Chem.* (U.S.S.R.), **28**, 2320 (1958); **29**, 1706 (1959).
27. E. OCHIAI, T. OKAMOTO, S. SAKAI, T. SUGASAWA, and T. ONOUCHI, *Chem. and Pharm. Bull.*, **7**, 542 (1959).
28. K. WIESNER, S. ITO, and Z. VALENTA, *Experientia*, **14**, 167 (1958).
29. T. SUGASAWA, *Chem. and Pharm. Bull.*, **14**, 6 (1956); **9**, 889, 897 (1961).
30. H. A. D. JOWETT, *J. Chem. Soc.*, 1518 (1896).
31. A. LAWSON and J. E. C. TOPPS, *J. Chem. Soc.*, 1640 (1937).
32. W. A. JACOBS, *J. Org. Chem.*, **16**, 1593 (1951).
33. S. W. PELLETIER and W. A. JACOBS, *J. Amer. Chem. Soc.*, **76**, 4496 (1954).
34. C. F. HUEBNER and W. A. JACOBS, *J. Biol. Chem.*, **170**, 515 (1947).

35. C. F. HUEBNER and W. A. JACOBS, *J. Biol. Chem.*, **174**, 1001 (1948).
36. S. W. PELLETIER and W. A. JACOBS, *J. Amer. Chem. Soc.*, **78**, 4139 (1956).
37. W. A. JACOBS and L. C. CRAIG, *J. Biol. Chem.*, **147**, 567 (1943).
38. S. W. PELLETIER and W. A. JACOBS, *J. Amer. Chem. Soc.*, **78**, 4144 (1956).
39. S. W. PELLETIER and P. C. PARTHASARTHY, *J. Amer. Chem. Soc.*, **87**, 777 (1965).
40. W. A. JACOBS and L. C. CRAIG, *J. Biol. Chem.*, **143**, 589 (1942).
41. C. A. HUEBNER and W. A. JACOBS, *J. Biol. Chem.*, **170**, 203 (1947).
42. D. M. LOCKE and S. W. PELLETIER, *J. Amer. Chem. Soc.*, **80**, 2588 (1958); **81**, 2246 (1959).
43. D. DVORNIK and O. E. EDWARDS, *Chem. and Ind.*, 623 (1958).
44. J. W. APSIMON and O. E. EDWARDS, *Canad. J. Chem.*, **40**, 896 (1962).
45. S. W. PELLETIER, *Chem. and Ind.*, 1116 (1958).
46. S. W. PELLETIER, *J. Amer. Chem. Soc.*, **82**, 2398 (1960).
47. S. W. PELLETIER and D. M. LOCKE, *J. Amer. Chem. Soc.*, **87**, 761 (1965).
48. D. DVORNIK and O. E. EDWARDS, *Chem. and Ind.*, 952 (1957); *Canad. J. Chem.*, **42**, 137 (1964).
49. O. E. EDWARDS and R. HOWE, *Proc. Chem. Soc.*, 62 (1959).
50. J. W. APSIMON, O. E. EDWARDS and R. HOWE, *Canad. J. Chem.*, **40**, 630 (1962).
51. S. W. PELLETIER and W. A. JACOBS, *Chem. and Ind.*, 1385 (1955).
52. O. E. EDWARDS and T. SINGH, *Canad. J. Chem.*, **32**, 465 (1954).
53. S. W. PELLETIER, *Chem. and Ind.*, 1016 (1956); 1670 (1957).
54. S. W. PELLETIER, *J. Amer. Chem. Soc.*, **87**, 799 (1965).
55. D. HUNTER, *Quart. J. Pharm.*, **17**, 302 (1944).
56. J. A. GOODSON, *J. Chem. Soc.*, 245 (1945).
57. D. DVORNIK and O. E. EDWARDS, *Tetrahedron*, **14**, 54 (1961).
58. D. DVORNIK and O. E. EDWARDS, *Proc. Chem. Soc.*, 280 (1958).
59. D. DVORNIK and O. E. EDWARDS, *Proc. Chem. Soc.*, 305 (1958).
60. E. OCHIAI, T. OKAMOTO, T. SUGASAWA, H. TANI and H. S. HAI, *J. Pharm. Soc.* (Japan), **72**, 816, 1605 (1952).
61. E. OCHIAI, T. OKAMOTA, S. SAKAI, M. KANEKO, K. FUJISAWA, V. NAGAI and H. TANI, *J. Pharm. Soc.* (Japan), **76**, 550 (1956).
62. E. OCHIAI, T. OKAMOTA, T. SUGASAWA, H. TANI, S. SAKAI, H. S. HAI and H. ENDO, *Chem. and Pharm. Bull.*, **1**, 60 (1953).
63. E. OCHIAI and T. OKAMOTO, *Chem. and Pharm. Bull.*, **7**, 550 (1959).
64. E. OCHIAI, T. OKAMOTO, T. SUGASAWA and S. SAKAI, *Chem. and Pharm. Bull.*, **2**, 388 (1954).
65. E. OCHIAI, T. OKAMOTO, S. HARA, S. SAKAI, and M. NATSUME, *Chem. and Pharm. Bull.*, **6**, 327 (1958).
66. E. OCHIAI, T. OKAMOTO, T. SUGASAWA, H. TANI and S. SAKAI, *Chem. and Pharm. Bull.*, **1**, 152 (1953).
67. S. SAKAI, *Chem. and Pharm. Bull.*, **6**, 448 (1958); **7**, 50, 55 (1959).
68. M. NATSUME, *Chem. and Pharm. Bull.*, **8**, 374 (1960).
69. T. OKAMOTO, *Chem. and Pharm. Bull.*, **7**, 44 (1959).
70. H. SUGINOME and F. SHIMANOUCHI, *Ann.*, **545**, 220 (1940).
71. M. NATSUME, *Chem. and Pharm. Bull.*, **10**, 879 (1962).
72. T. OKAMOTO, M. NATSUME, H. ZENDA, and S. KAMATA, *Chem. and Pharm. Bull.*, **10**, 883 (1962).
73. W. A. JACOBS and L. C. CRAIG, *J. Biol. Chem.*, **143**, 605 (1942).
74. M. H. BENN, *Canad. J. Chem.*, **44**, 1 (1966).
75. M. PRZYBYLSKA, *Canad. J. Chem.*, **40**, 566 (1962).
76. K. WIESNER, Z. VALENTA and L. G. HUMBER, *Tetrahedron Letters*, 621 (1962).

CHAPTER 6

THE ACONITE ALKALOIDS

THE aconitines form a series of highly toxic ester-bases isolated from both *Aconitum* and *Delphinium* species. Aconite root (derived mainly from *A. napellus*) formerly found some use in folk-medicine. The diterpenoid C-19 alkamine or basic fragment (aconine) is esterified with acids such as acetic, benzoic or veratric acids. The biogenesis of the parent C-19 skeleton (I) may lie through compounds of the atisine skeleton (II). This would involve loss of C-17, a Wagner–Meerwein rearrangement of the C-8–C-9 bond possibly facilitated by an equatorial leaving group at C-15, and a cyclization from C-20. The alkamine fragments then fall into two groups: those resembling lycoctonine (III) in possessing a 7-hydroxyl and those resembling aconine (IV) which lack this feature. The parent alkamines can then be classified as follows:

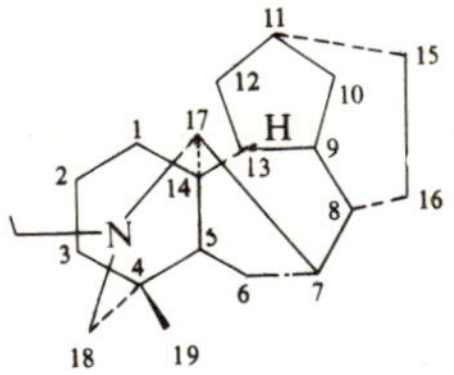

I

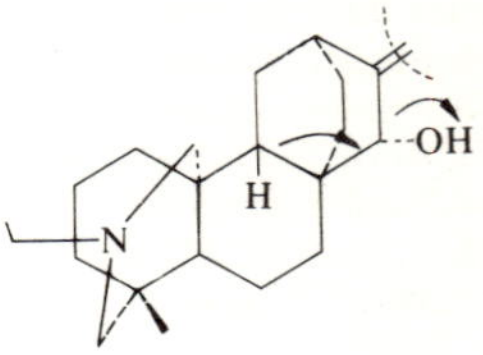

II

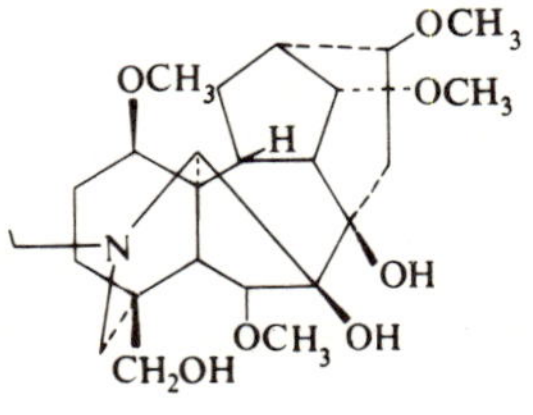

III

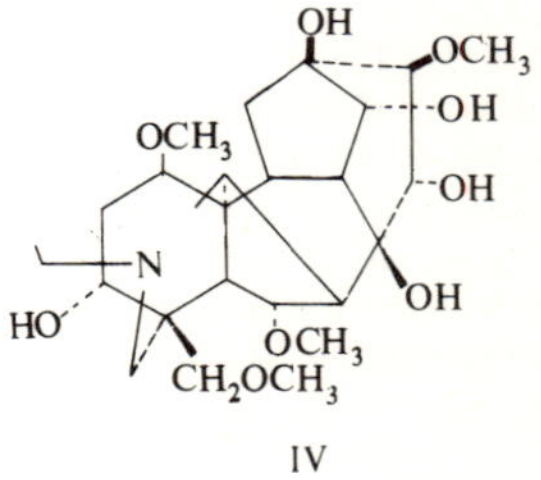

IV

Lycoctonines	*Aconines*
Browniine	Aconine
Delcosine	Bikhaconine
Delpheline	Chasmanine
Delsoline	Delphonine
Lycoctonine	Pseudoaconine

Heteroatisine forms a lactonic derivative related to the aconines. The esterifying aromatic acids are usually attached to the alkamine at position 10 whilst a hydroxyl at position 8 may often be acetylated.

Whilst a considerable chemical effort has been devoted to the study of these alkaloids, many of their reactions have only recently been rationalized in terms of structures derived from X-ray analysis. Indeed this field clearly illustrates the value of such studies. Thus although aconitine was isolated about 1860 and its simpler derivatives characterized in 1875, the chemistry of the group was not placed on a rational basis until the late 1950's. Much of the earlier work was concerned with the differential reactivity of the several hydroxyl groups. The analytical data was complicated by the tendency of the molecules to solvate. Although oxidation and pyrolysis experiments gave valuable evidence for the relative disposition of the various oxygen substituents, they were less clear cut as regards defining the carbon skeleton, dehydrogenation experiments were of little value and at one stage misleading. The key member of this series is the alkamine lycoctonine and its chemistry will therefore be described first. A number of reviews have been devoted to the chemistry of these alkaloids.[1-3]

6.1. *Lycoctonine*

The alkaloid lycoctonine (III) $C_{25}H_{41}O_7N$ occurs as its free base and as its esters with anthranilic acid, *N*-acetylanthranilic acid, *N*-succinylanthranilic acid, and *N*-methylsuccinylanthranilic acid in a number of *Aconitum* and *Delphinium* species, such as *A. lycoctonum*,[4] *D. ajacis*,[5] *D. barbeyi*,[6] and *D. elatum*.[7] It has also been isolated[8,9] from *Inula royleana*, a member of the *Compositae*.

After considerable chemical degradation, the structure and absolute configuration were determined[10] by an X-ray analysis of des(oxymethylene)-lycoctonine (V). The chemistry of lycoctonine has now been rationalized in these terms and a biogenetic relationship to atisine proposed.[11,12]

The alkaloid was characterized as a tertiary base [pK_a^{12} 8·8 in 50 per cent aqueous methanol] containing an *N*-ethyl group. The oxygen functions were accounted for by four methoxy and three hydroxyl groups to which the various ester groupings were attached.[13] The base was saturated and hence it was hexacyclic. Much of the earlier work involved oxidative evidence which served to establish the nature of four out of the six rings and to locate six of the eight substituents.

Oxidation[14] with chromium trioxide involved preferential attack on the primary hydroxyl group to form an aldehyde lycoctonal (VI). Wolff–Kishner reduction of this aldehyde then gave deoxylycoctonine. On the other hand oxidation with potassium permanganate gave two neutral lactams – oxolycoctonine (lycoctonam) (VII; R = CH_2OH) and desoxymethylenelycoctonam (VII; R = H) together with an acid, lycoctonamic acid (VII; R = CO_2H). Both lycoctonam and the methyl ester of lycoctonamic acid were reduced with lithium aluminium hydride to lycoctonine thus eliminating the possibility of skeletal change during the oxidation. The acid underwent decarboxylation to form desoxymethylenelycoctonam. This evidence required the presence of the grouping $\rangle N-CH_2-\overset{|}{\underset{|}{C}}-C-CH_2OH$ in lycocotine. Furthermore, the lactam infrared absorption (in the range 1590–1630 cm^{-1}) implied the location of the nitrogen in a six-membered or larger ring.

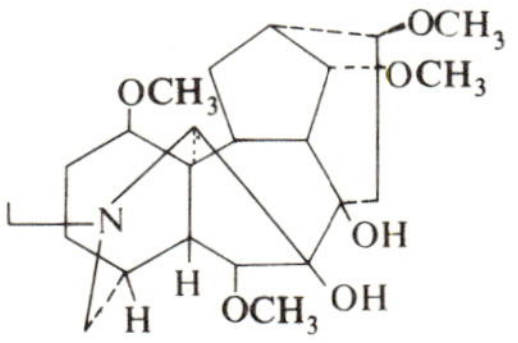

V

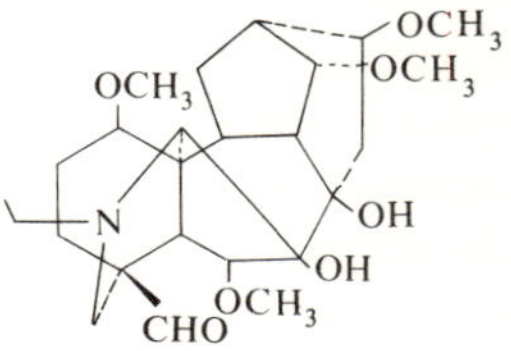

VI

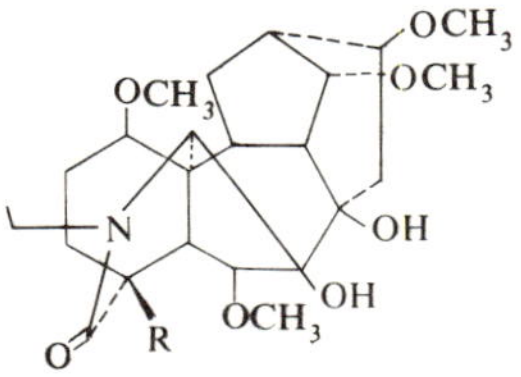

VII

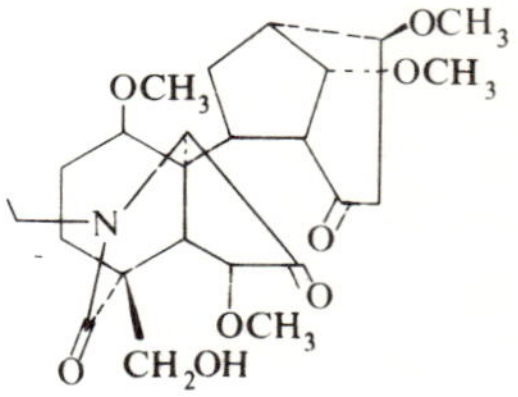

VIII

Evidence for the existence of a ditertiary α-glycol in lycoctonine came[15–17] from the reaction of periodic acid with lycoctonam and the formation of diketone (VIII). Similarly, cleavage of desoxymethylenelycoctonam also gave a diketone. The infrared spectra (ν_{max} 1766, 1707, and 1631 cm^{-1} and 1765, 1707, 1644 cm^{-1} respectively) indicated the generation of a cyclopentanone and a cyclohexanone. Both diketones could be reduced catalytically or with sodium borohydride to give ketols in which the cyclopentanone had been reduced. Both diketones show an unusual ultraviolet spectrum with a high end-absorption and a maximum at 318 mμ (log ϵ 2·45) and 322 mμ (log ϵ 2·42) respectively which is absent from the ultraviolet spectrum of the ketols. This reflects a transannular interaction with nitrogen of the heterocyclic ring.

The diketones, but not the ketols, reduced Tollens' reagent and Fehling's solution and hence a further oxygen function (a methoxyl group) was located adjacent to the cyclopentanone. Furthermore, treatment of both the diketones and ketols with acid or alkali resulted in the loss of methanol and the formation of an $\alpha\beta$-unsaturated ketone (λ_{max} 223 mμ; ν_{max} 1679 cm^{-1}). Hence a methoxyl occupied the β-position to the cyclohexanone.

Mildly basic conditions (e.g. activated alumina or sodium bicarbonate) served[17] to convert the diketone (VIII) to an isomer involving the loss of the cyclohexanone and the generation of a new tertiary hydroxyl group. The product was formulated as (IX) resulting from an internal aldol condensation. Treatment of this isomer with hot 6N acid, gave a mixture consisting of an "α-iso" compound, $C_{25}H_{37}O_8N$, (X) and an "anhydro-iso" compound, $C_{25}H_{35}O_7N$, (XI). The former no longer contained a primary alcohol whilst its two hydroxyl functions behaved as hindered tertiary alcohols. The second product which lacked hydroxyl absorption [(ν_{max} 1736 cm^{-1})] was ketonic and contained the abnormal ultraviolet absorption noted previously (λ_{max} 300 mμ, log ϵ 1·9). It was therefore formulated as the product of a pinacolic rearrangement. A related rearrangement occurred[18] on treatment of lycoctonam with acetyl chloride. The product, anhydrolycoctonam acetate was hydrolysed by base to anhydrolycoctonam (XII). The desoxymethylene series underwent a similar isomerization to form anhydrodesoxymethylenelycoctonam.

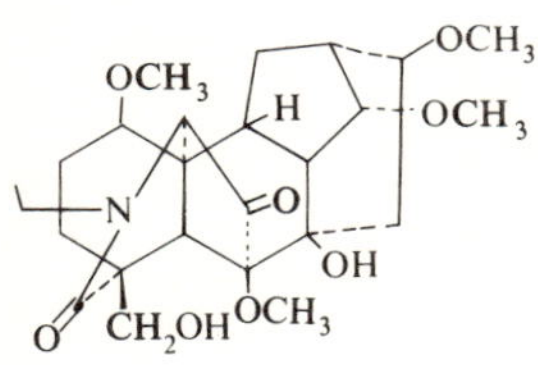

IX

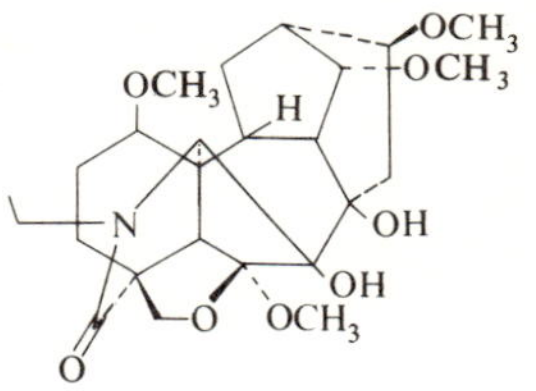

X

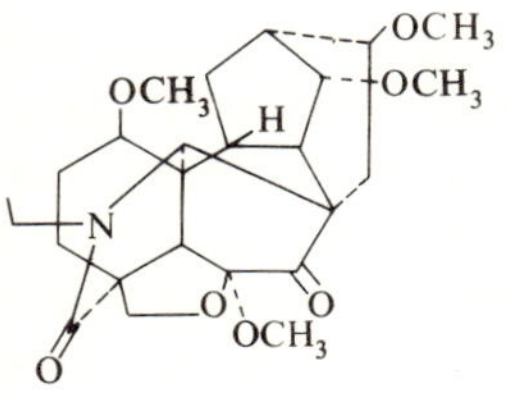

XI

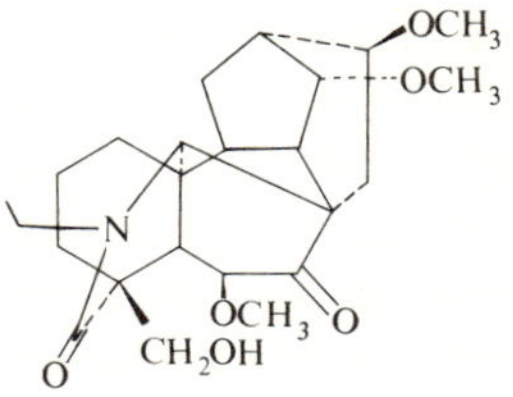

XII

Lycoctonine is readily oxidized[19,21] by silver oxide to hydroxylycoctonine, $C_{25}H_{41}O_8N$. The structure of this carbinolamine ether has been defined as (XIII) on the basis of an X-ray analysis Hydroxylycoctonine forms a series of anhydronium bases suggesting the presence of an additional oxygen atom adjacent to the nitrogen. However, structures such as (XIV) for these bases derived from (XV) involve violation of Bredt's rule. Catalytic reduction of hydroxylycoctonine gave a ketonic isomer of lycoctonine (isolycoctonine) by hydrogenolysis of the ether ring.

On oxidation with potassium permanganate hydroxylycoctonine gave a series of lactams. Similar oxidation of isolycoctonine with lead tetra-acetate resulted[21] in a lactam which was further oxidized to a keto-acid (XVI). The carboxylic acid formed a lactone with the primary hydroxyl

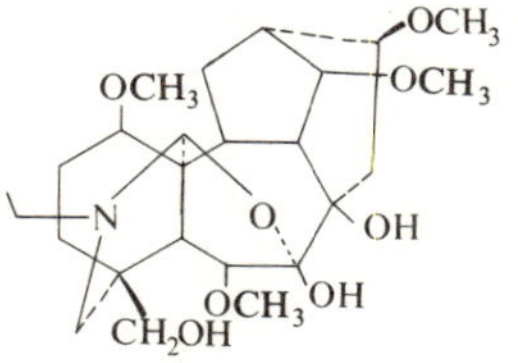

XIII

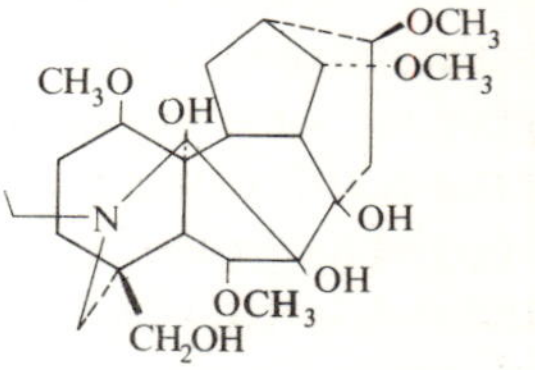

XIV

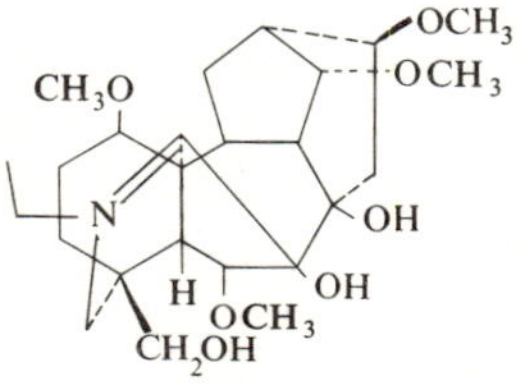

XV

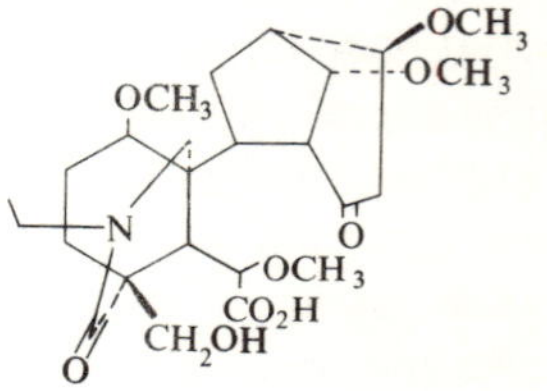

XVI

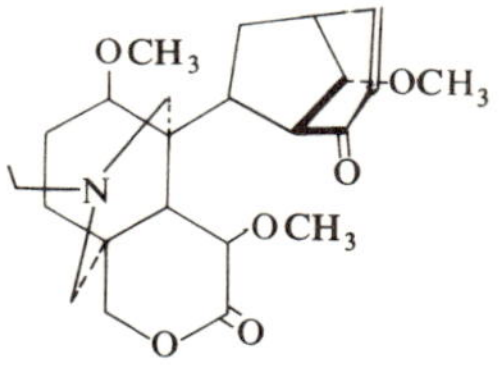

XVII

and on treatment with dilute acid lost the elements of methanol to give an $\alpha\beta$-unsaturated ketone (XVII). Furthermore, treatment of isolycoctonam with zinc and acetic acid led to the elimination of the 8-hydroxyl. This product on further treatment with sodium amalgam lost the 6-methoxyl group. These degradations which were of value in determining the structure of hydroxylycoctonine, established a 1:5 relationship between the 18-hydroxyl group and the carbonyl group of hydroxylycoctonine together with the ring B substitution pattern.

6.2. *Delpheline*

Delpheline, methyl lycaconitine and deltaline were isolated[5] from *Delphinium elatum*. Preliminary characterization indicated that delpheline (XVIII), $C_{25}H_{39}O_6N$, contained three methoxyls and a methylenedioxy group together with an *N*-ethyl group. Much of the chemistry of the delpheline resembles that of lycoctonine. The *N*-ethyl group was removed by oxidation with mercuric acetate to form α-hydroxydelpheline, in turn oxidized with potassium permanganate to the *N*-acetyl derivative and hydrolysed by acid to des-ethyldelpheline. Alternatively, nitrosation and hydrogenolysis gave the des-ethyl derivative directly.

Oxidation[22] of delpheline with potassium permanganate in acetone or with chromium trioxide in pyridine yielded the neutral lactam, oxodelpheline, whose infrared spectrum possessed carbonyl absorption indicative of a six-membered lactam. On the other hand oxidation of delpheline with chromium trioxide in acetic acid, *N*-bromosuccinimide, or silver oxide, gave a cyclopentanone, dehydrodelpheline. This ketone lacked further hydroxylic absorption and hence the remaining oxygen atoms were ethereal. These oxidations could be reversed by reduction with lithium aluminium hydride with the regeneration of delpheline.

Treatment of delpheline and its oxidation products with strong acid led to the liberation of formaldehyde and the generation of a diol. Since demethylene-delpheline consumed two moles of lead tetra-acetate and dehydrodemethylene-oxodelpheline consumed only one mole whilst the

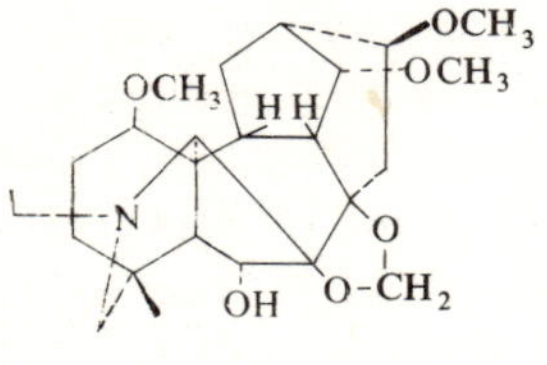

XVIII

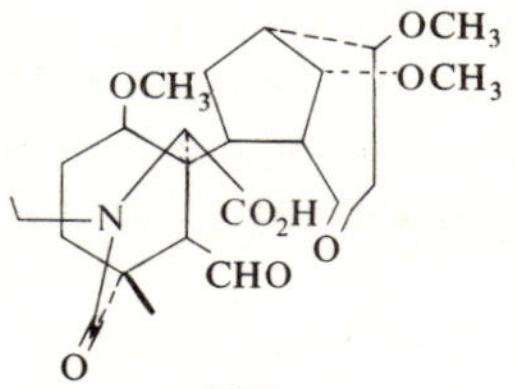

XIX

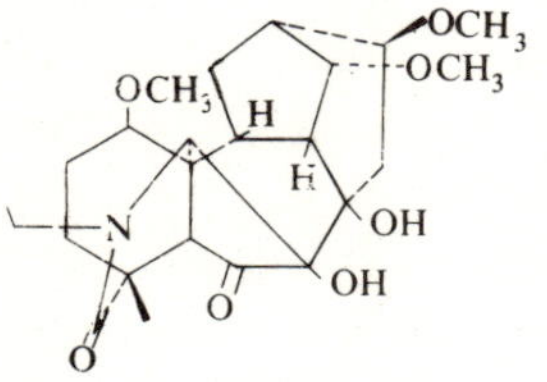

XX

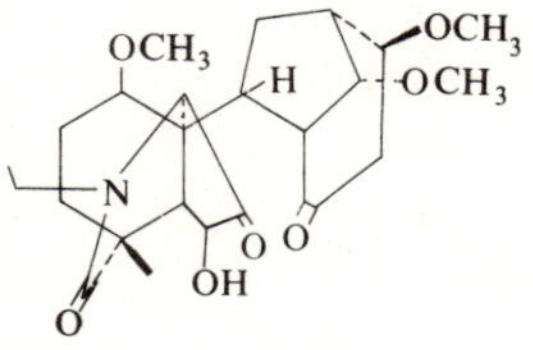

XXI

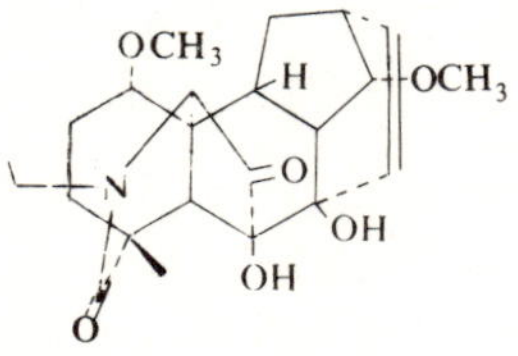

XXII

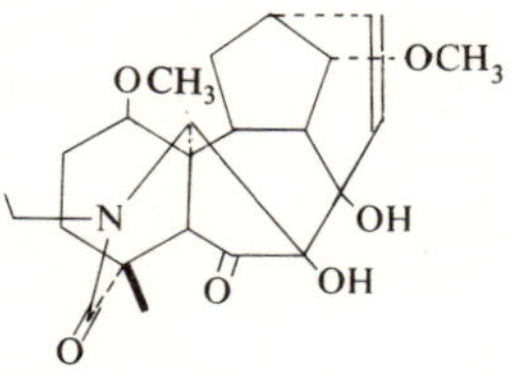

XXIII

parent delpheline was inert, this hydrolysis product, demethylenedelpheline contains a 1,2,3-triol. Thus careful oxidation[23,24] of demethylene-oxodelpheline with one mole of periodic acid yielded a diketone containing an additional cyclopentanone (ν_{max} 1754 cm^{-1}) and a cyclohexanone (ν_{max} 1710 cm^{-1}) typical of the oxidation of a ditertiary glycol. Further oxidation of this seco-diketone with alkaline periodate yielded a diseco-acid-aldehyde (XIX). This clearly defined the presence of a 1,2,3-triol. β-Elimination of methanol from this acid gave an $\alpha\beta$-unsaturated ketone.

Oxidation of the lactam (XX) with lead tetra-acetate led to cleavage of the α-glycol and to the formation of a cyclopentanedione and a cyclohexanone. Interestingly this compound and its relatives are red in colour. The diketone (XXI) and its $\alpha\beta$-unsaturated relative underwent a base-catalysed aldol condensation to form (XXII) (or (XXIII)). The former is analogous to the isolycoctonine series whilst the latter contains the original ring system.

Deoxymethylenedelpheline on vigorous treatment with acetyl chloride undergoes a pinacol rearrangement to form the ketol acetate (XXIV) analogous to the rearrangement of anhydrolycoctonine.

In view of the evident relationship with lycoctonine an experimental link between the two series was provided[24] by the transformation of lycoctonine to the ketone (XXV). Reduction with sodium amalgam led to the elimination of the 6-methoxyl group. Subsequent oxidation with selenium dioxide then led to the α-diketone (XXVI) derived from delpheline.

Deltaline has been related[23] by dehydration and hydrogenation to acetyldelpheline.

XXIV

XXV

XXVI

6.3. *Delcosine and Delsoline*

Delcosine (XXVII), $C_{24}H_{39}O_7N$, isolated[7] from *Delphinium consolida*, is identical[30] to Alkaloid C (from *D. elatum*[5]), delphamine,[1,25] Takaobase-I,[26] and lucaconine (from *Aconitum lucidusculum*).[27–29] whilst its monoacetyl derivative[28] is alkaloid B (from *D. elatum*[5]). Dehydrodelcosine is Shimoburobase-II. Delsoline, $C_{25}H_{41}O_7N$, was isolated[7] also from *Delphinium consolida*.

Delcosine contained[24,31] four hydroxyl groups, two of which are secondary and readily acetylated, and three methoxyl groups. On the other hand delsoline contained three hydroxyl groups and four methoxyl groups. Their close relationship was demonstrated[30] as delcosine on methylation with sodium hydride and methyl iodide formed delsoline. Oxidation of delcosine with chromium trioxide gave a diketo-lactam containing both a cyclopentanone and a cyclohexanone whilst oxidation of delsoline gave only a monoketo-lactam. On the other hand Oppenauer oxidation of delcosine gave dehydrodelcosine containing a cyclopentanone. The absence of a big change in pK_a indicated that the ring D hydroxyl had been oxidized. The relationship of the hydroxyl groups in delcosine was established by the consumption of 5 moles periodate indicating a vicinal triol whilst ether formation established the presence of a further free hydroxyl at C-18. The anhydro base then consumed only one mole of periodate. The existence of a ditertiary α-glycol in delsoline was established[32,33] by cleavage with periodate. An attempt[34] to chemically relate the carbon skeleton to that of lycoctonine was unsuccessful and recourse was made[35] to X-ray analysis for a solution to the problem.

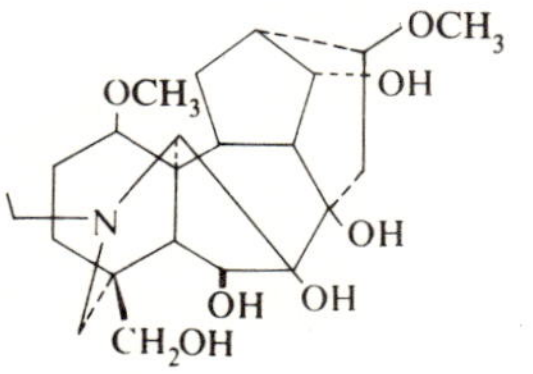

XXVII

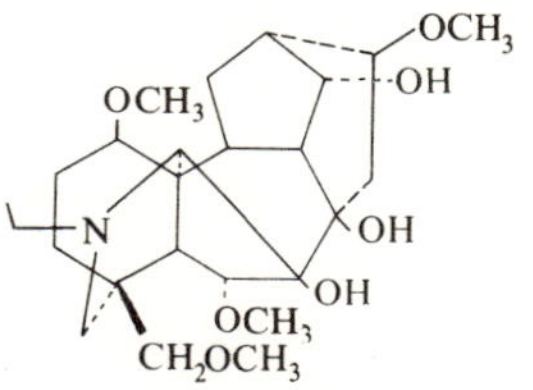

XXVIII

6.4. *Browniine*

Browniine (XXVIII) and its 16-dehydro derivative which fall into this group of bases, were isolated[36,37] from *Delphinium cardinale*. Lead tetraacetate oxidation of browniine gave a 7–20 ether comparable with hydroxylycoctonine. This was in turn related to the alkamine chasmanine of known structure.

6.5. *Aconitine*

Aconitine is the principal alkaloid[38] of *Aconitum napellus* and occurs widely[1] in other *Aconitum* species. It is one of the most readily accessible of the Aconite alkaloids and unfortunately it is also one of the most complex. Its confusing and often contradictory chemistry has been reviewed[1-3] on a number of occasions. Aconine (XXIX) is the parent alkamine of aconitine (the acetate, benzoate) and jesaconitine[39,40] (the acetate, *p*-methoxybenzoate). Aconine is closely related to mesaconine[41,42] which is the *N*-methyl rather than the *N*-ethyl analogue.

The alkaloid was first isolated[38] about 1860 and characterized[43] in 1875. Many subsequent studies led[1] to a clarification of the functional groups as three hydroxyls, four methoxyls, an acetate, a benzoate and an *N*-ethyl group. The key to the structure of the alkaloid came from an X-ray

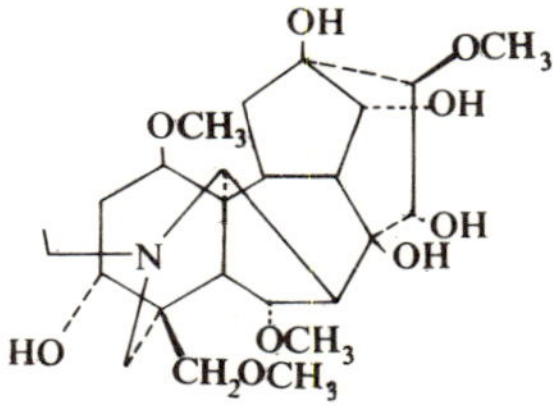

XXIX

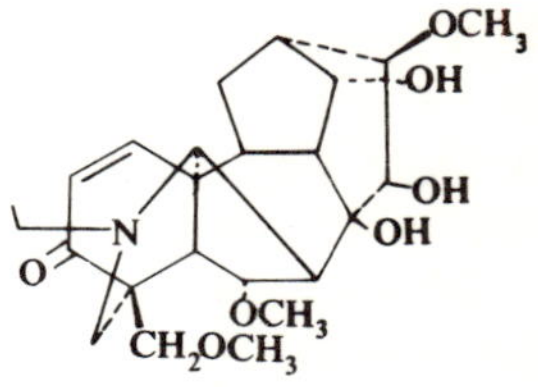

XXX

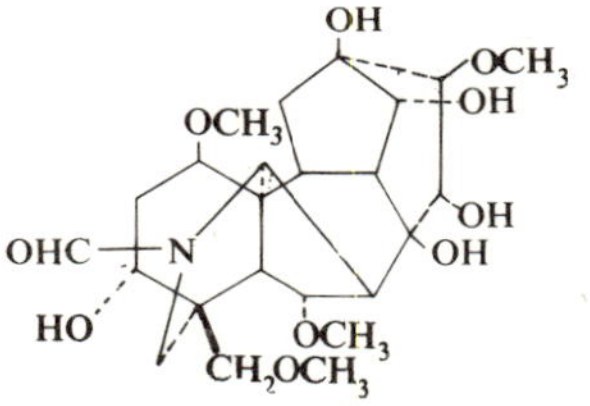

XXXI

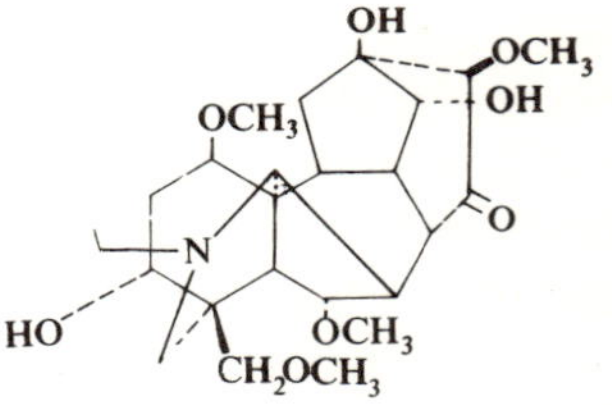

XXXII

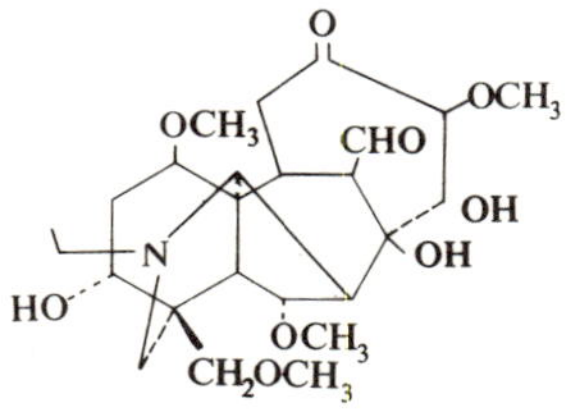

XXXIII

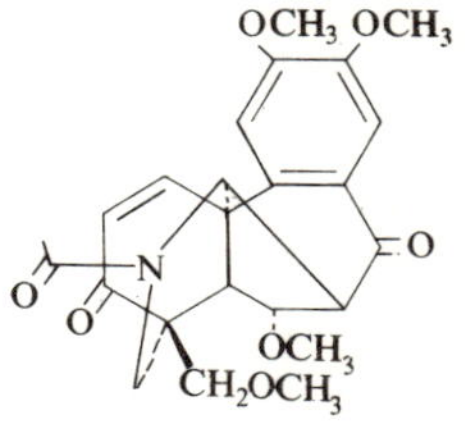

XXXIV

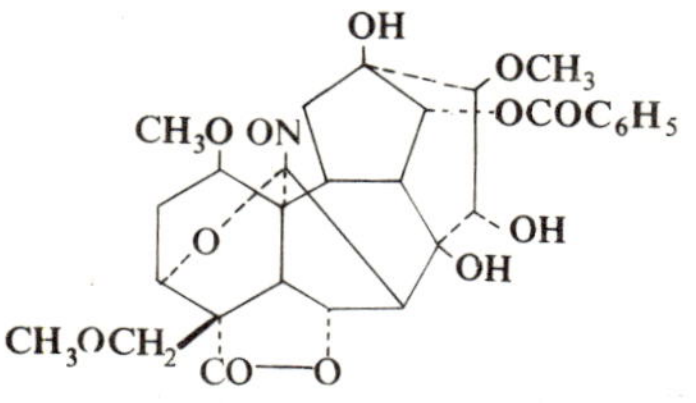

XXXV

analysis[44] of the oxidation product,[45] aconinone hydrobromide. Independent chemical evidence led[46] simultaneously to the same conclusion and this was further extended[47] to clarify the structure of ring A.

The major degradative reactions[48, 49] of aconitine can be exemplified as follows. Oxidation[45] with chromium trioxide gives a ring A ketone which loses methanol to give the $\alpha\beta$-unsaturated ketone, aconitoline. This may in turn be hydrolysed to aconinone (XXX). On the other hand the primary product of oxidation with potassium permanganate is a product of dealkylation, oxonitine. The corresponding alkamine, oxonine, has been repeatedly investigated and eventually shown[50, 51] to be the *N*-formyl derivative (XXXI). Oxidation with nitric acid appears to be more complex[49] forming a nitronitroso-compound, $C_{31}H_{35}O_{13}N_3$.

Pyrolysis of the alkaloid leads to the elimination of acetic acid and the formation of pyraconitine[52] which on alkaline hydrolysis affords benzoic acid and pyraconine (XXXII). In this case the elimination of the tertiary acetate characteristic of lycoctonine and delpheline chemistry, has resulted in the formation of a ketone. Wolff–Kishner reduction of this α-methoxyketone afforded an olefin in turn obtained[53] from pseudoaconine. A direct relationship has also been established[54] between delphinine and aconitine. Thus cleavage of oxonine (XXXI) with 1 mole of periodate led to an aldehyde (XXXIII) which with alkali undergoes a pinacolic rearrangement and aromatization to a phenol. The corresponding methyl ether was characterized as its oxidation product (XXXIV). A similar aromatic ether was prepared from both aconitine and delphinine forming a link which served to establish the identity of the ring A methoxyl in both alkaloids. The stereochemistry of ring A was determined through the formation of nitroso lactones containing an ether link (XXXV) whose formation requires the presence of a hydroxyl and angular function on the same side of the molecule.

6.6. *Pseudoaconitine*

Pseudoaconitine, $C_{36}H_{51}O_{12}N$, was isolated[55] in 1878 from *Aconitum ferox* (*deinorrhizum*) and subsequently from *A. balfourii*, *A. napellus*, and *A. spicatum*.[1, 56, 57, 58] It was hydrolysed to an alkamine pseudoaconine (XXXVI) together with acetic and veratric acids. Pseudoaconine also formed the alkamine of indaconitine[59] (from *A. chasmanthum*) in which it is esterified with acetic and benzoic acids. Its structure was established by the conversion[60] of indaconitine to delphinine in which the ring A hydroxyl was removed. The alkaloid was also related[61] to aconitine. Thus pseudoaconitine was converted to a pyroderivative, in which the double bond was then isomerized to form demethoxyisopyropseudoaconine (XXXVII). This was identical to the Wolff–Kishner reduction product of pyraconitine.

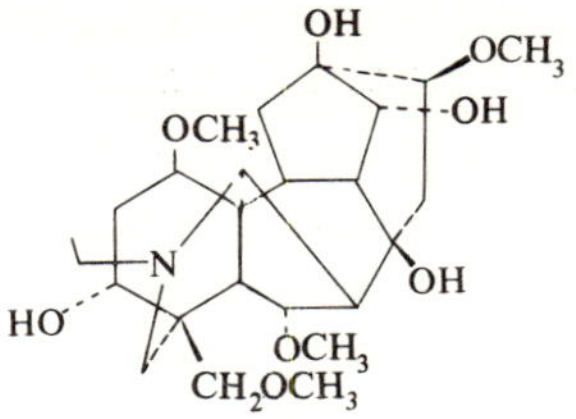

XXXVI

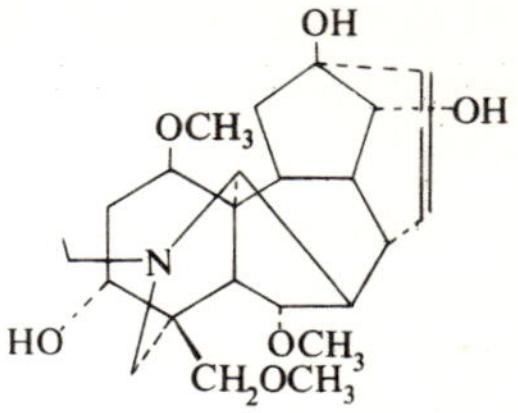

XXXVII

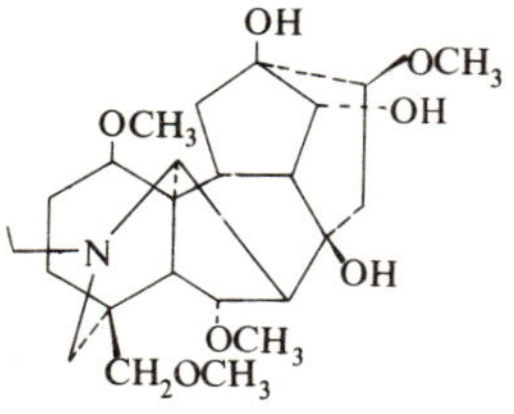

XXXVIII

6.7. *Bikhaconine*

Bikhaconite, isolated[62] from *Aconitum spicatum*, is the veratric acid ester of bikhaconine (XXXVIII). The benzoate is chasmaconitine[59] (from *A. chasmanthum*) and the cinnamate, chasmanthinine. The structure[63, 64] of bikhaconine rests upon a relationship with pseudoaconitine in which the ring A hydroxyl of the latter was eliminated.

6.8. *Chasmanine*

Chasmanine (XXXIX) (from *A. chasmanthum* and *A. subcuneatum*) was shown[65] to contain an *N*-ethyl group, four methoxyl groups and two hydroxyls. Oxidation characterized one of these as a secondary hydroxyl

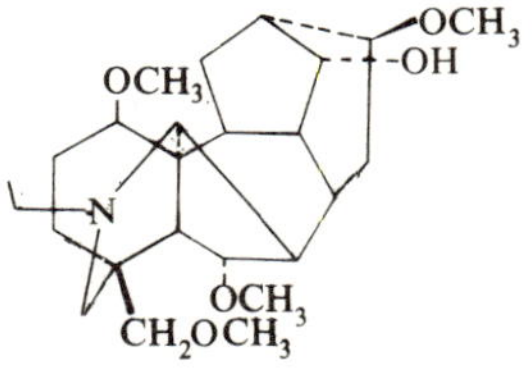

XXXIX

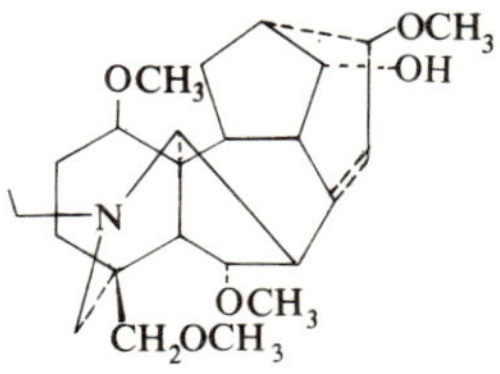

XL

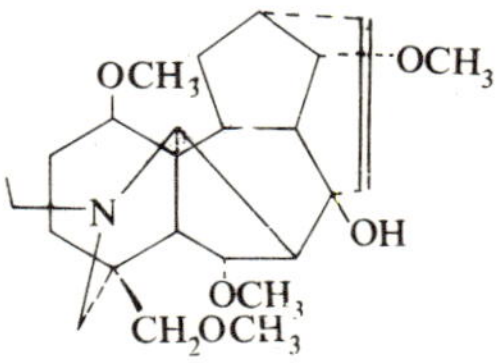

XLI

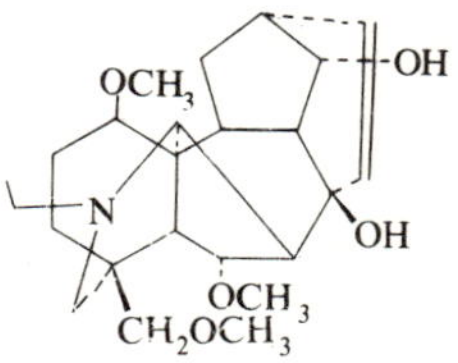

XLII

group on a five membered ring. Chasmanine underwent the pyrolytic reactions typical of the fragment $\gt C{\cdot}OH{\cdot}CH_2{\cdot}CH(OCH_3)$. Three compounds were isolated from this pyrolysis, pyrochasmanine (XL), isopyrochasmanine (XLI) and demethylisopyrochasmanine (XLII).

The n.m.r. spectra of the acetoxy-benzoate clarified the position and stereochemistry of the ring D hydroxyl which from the multiplicity of the resonance, was flanked by two hydrogens. The alkaloid has been correlated[66] with browniine (XXVIII).

6.9. *Condelphine, Isotalatizidine, Talatizidine*

Condelphine (XLIII) has been isolated[1,67] from *Delphinium confusum* and *D. denudatum*. The parent amino-alcohol is identical to isotalatizi-

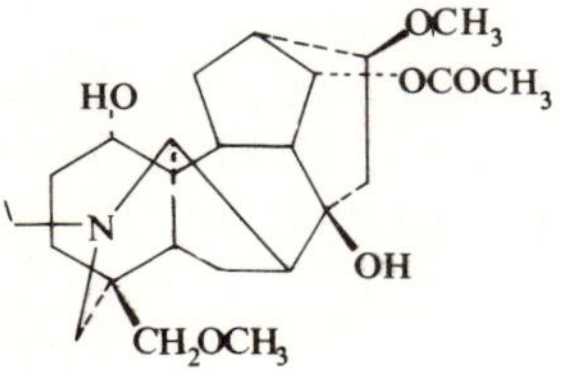

HO; OCH3; OCOCH3; N; OH; CH2OCH3

XLIII

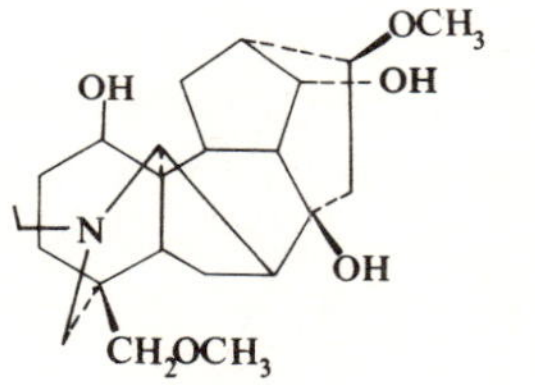

OH; OCH3; OH; N; OH; CH2OCH3

XLIV

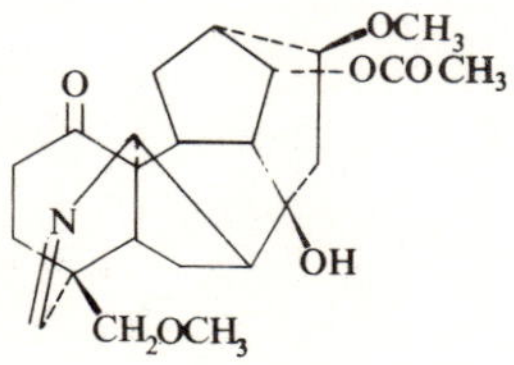

O; OCH3; OCOCH3; N; OH; CH2OCH3

XLV

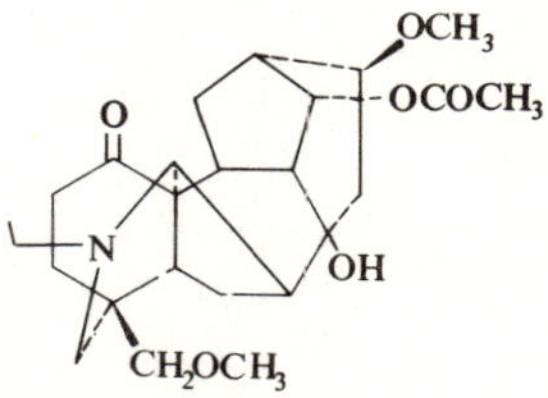

O; OCH3; OCOCH3; N; OH; CH2OCH3

XLVI

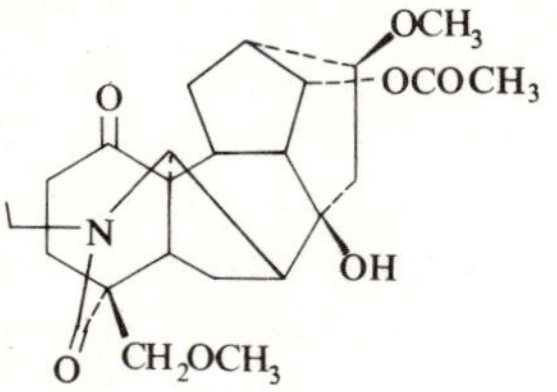

O; OCH3; OCOCH3; N; OH; O; CH2OCH3

XLVII

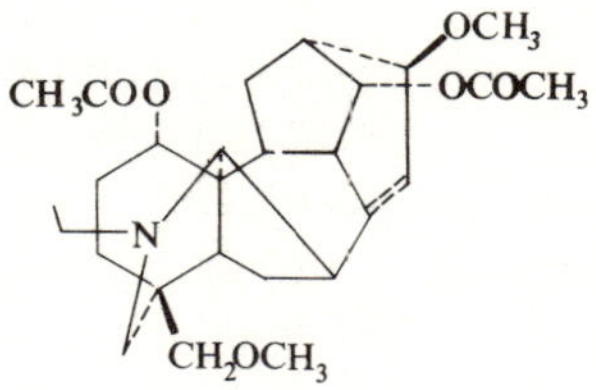

CH3COO; OCH3; OCOCH3; N; CH2OCH3

XLVIII

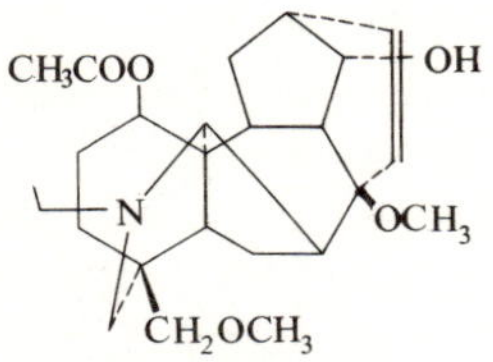

CH3COO; OH; N; OCH3; CH2OCH3

XLIX

dine from *Aconitum talissicum* whilst the 1-epimer with a β-hydroxyl is talatizidine (XLIV) from the same plant.

Oxidation of condelphine generated an imine (XLV), a ketone (XLVI) and a keto-lactam (XLVII). Reduction of the imine and reaction with ethyl iodide gave a mixture of talatizidine and isotalatizidine. The position of one of the methoxyl groups on the primary centre in condelphine was evident from the n.m.r. spectrum of the alkaloid and its ketonic derivatives. Evidence for the location of a hydroxyl group at C-1 came from its elimination reactions to give a single Δ^1-olefin with the expected n.m.r. spectrum. Furthermore, the triacetyl amino-alcohol underwent the typical "pyro" elimination reaction characteristic of these alkaloids to form (XLVIII) in turn isomerized to an isopyro (XLIX) derivative.

6.10. *Delphinine*

Delphinine is the principle alkaloid of *Delphinium staphisagria*.[1,68,69] On hydrolysis it yields benzoic acid, acetic acid and an alkamine delphonine (L), $C_{24}H_{39}O_7N$. The latter contains four methoxyl groups,[70] an *N*-methyl group, and three hydroxyl groups, two of which are tertiary and one secondary.

Oxidation of delphinine provided[71,72] two degradation products, an *N*-formyl derivative, α-oxodelphinine, and a δ-lactam, β-oxodelphinine. α-Oxodelphinine underwent pyrolytic loss of acetic acid to give pyro-α-oxodelphinine (LI). The isomerization of this isopyro-α-oxodelphinine is an allylic rearrangement involving exchange of a methoxyl with a solvent molecule. Exploration of the isopyro system indicated that it contained the fragment (LII) and that the benzoate of delphinine was attached to a secondary position on a cyclopentane ring. The corresponding dihydroketone (LIII) was capable of undergoing an acyloin rearrangement to (LIV) which may in turn be cleaved to a carboxylic acid. The elimination of methanol during this change clarified the substitution pattern of this portion of the ring system.

The extension of these partial formulae to a complete formula for delphinine then followed. A lycoctonine-type skeleton was initially assumed and its presence then rigorously demonstrated. The key to the disposition of the remaining three methoxyl groups came from some displacement experiments. The differing reactivity of the methoxyl groups enabled them to be distinguished. Two of the methoxyl groups of isopyro-α-oxodelphinine are reversibly displaced[71] by chlorine. Furthermore, zinc chloride will convert two of the methoxyl groups to a hydroxyl and the remaining two to a cyclic ether (LV). In the case of the latter one of the methoxyls involved in ether formation is a primary group which is also displaced by chlorine. Oxidation of the free ring A hydroxyl in (LV) gave a cyclohexanone and then a dibasic acid in which one carbonyl group was hindered.

Further evidence for the carbon skeleton came from the unusual Hofmann degradation product of delphonine. The genesis of the ketonic product (LVI) requires an initial 1:3 cleavage and then the disruption of rings C and D through a reverse aldol reaction, β-elimination of a methoxyl group and a vinylogous β-keto-aldehyde cleavage.

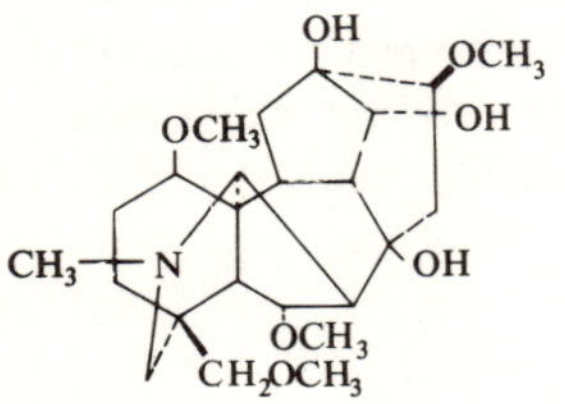

L

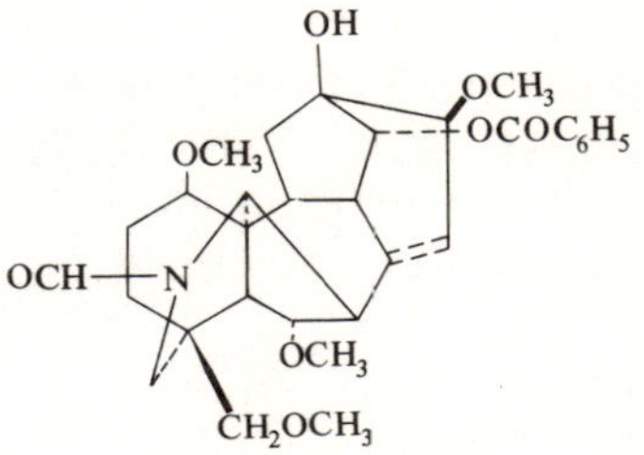

LI

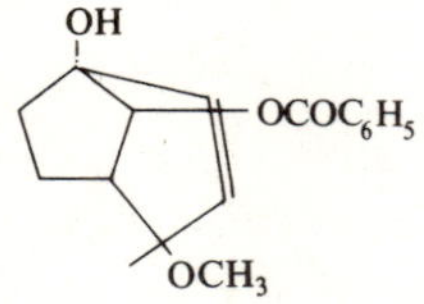

LII

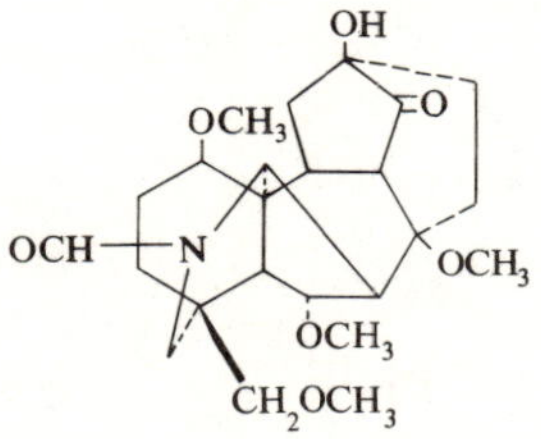

LIII

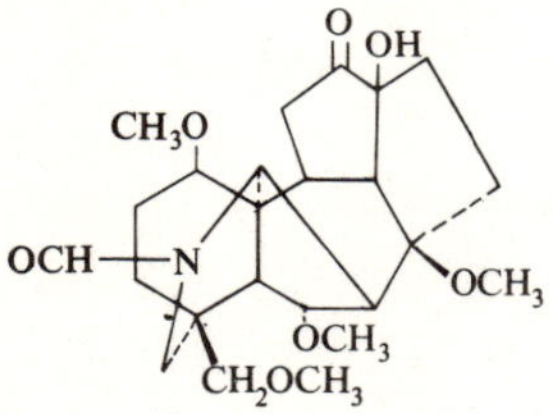

LIV

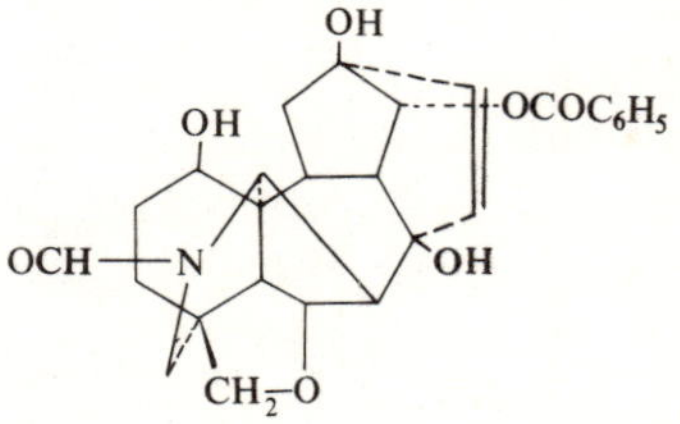

LV

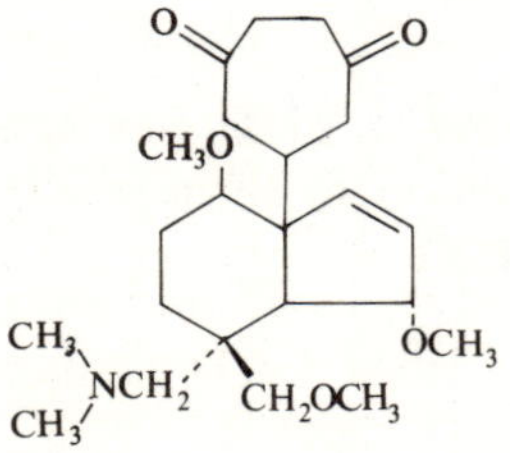

LVI

6.11. *Heteratisine*

Heteratisine is a lactonic alkaloid isolated[73] from *Aconitum heterophyllum*. Its structure (LVII) rests primarily on X-ray analysis[74] which received independent support[75, 76] from chemical degradation. The n.m.r. spectrum of the alkaloid indicated the presence of methoxyl, *N*-ethyl, *C*-methyl, a secondary hydroxyl and secondary lactonic hydroxyl functions, whilst the infrared spectrum showed carbonyl absorption typical of a δ-lactone. Chromium trioxide oxidation confirmed that one of the hydroxyl groups was secondary. Further oxidation gave a δ-lactam, oxoheteratisone. The relationship of the lactone ring, carbonyl and tertiary hydroxyl groups in the first oxidation product was evident from its decarboxylation in alkali involving a retroaldol reaction and subsequent decomposition of a β-keto-acid.

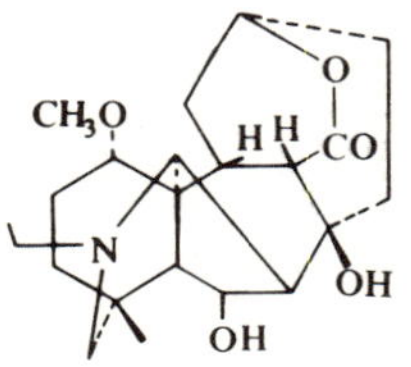

LVII

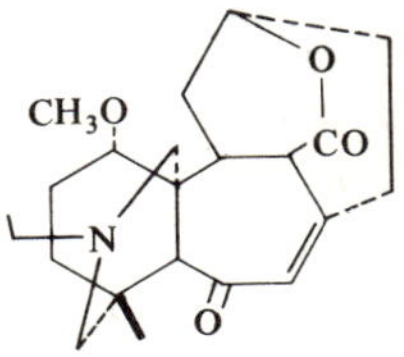

LVIII

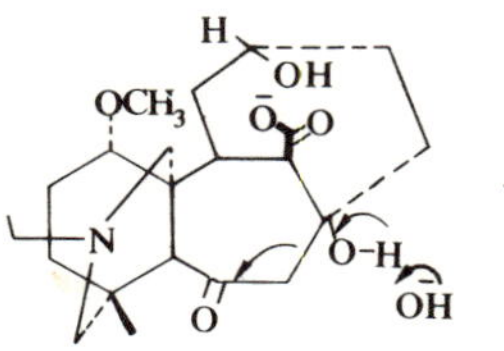

LIX

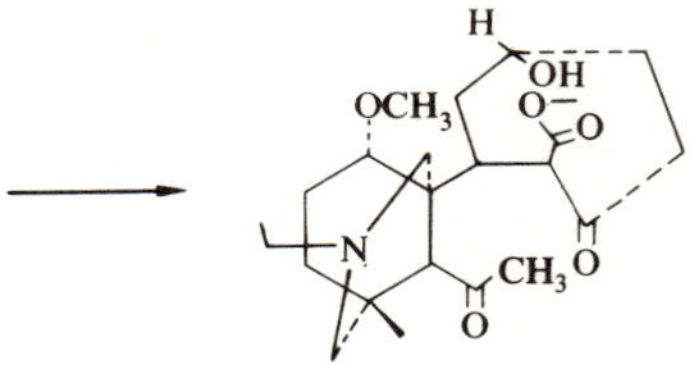

LX

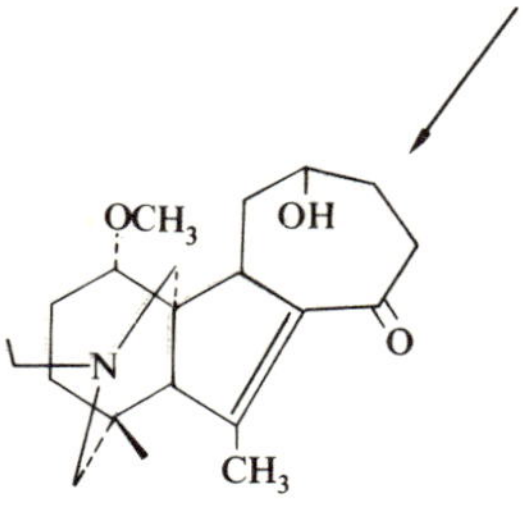

LXI

The nature of pyroheteratisine (LVIII) was apparent[77] from alkaline rearrangement and decarboxylation to form (LXI) presumably through the intervention of (LIX) and (LX).

REFERENCES

1. T. A. Henry, *The Plant Alkaloids*, p. 673, J. and A. Churchill, London (1949).
2. E. S. Stern in *The Alkaloids*, Ed. R. H. F. Manske, Vol. IV, p. 275, Academic Press, London (1954).

3. L. MARION, *I.U.P.A.C. Symposium*, Vol. 2, p. 621, Butterworths, London (1962).
4. H. SCHULZE and E. BIERLING, *Arch. Pharm.*, **251**, 8 (1913).
5. J. A. GOODSON, *J. Chem. Soc.*, 139 (1943); 108, 665 (1944); 245 (1945).
6. W. B. COOK and O. A. BEATH, *J. Amer. Chem. Soc.*, **74**, 1411 (1952).
7. L. MARION and O. E. EDWARDS, *J. Amer. Chem. Soc.*, **69**, 2010 (1947).
8. O. E. EDWARDS and M. N. RODGER, *Canad. J. Chem.*, **37**, 1187 (1959).
9. S. K. TALAPATRA and A. CHATTERJEE, *J. Indian Chem. Soc.*, **36**, 437
10. M. PRZYBYLSKA and L. MARION, *Canad. J. Chem.*, **34**, 185 (1956); **37**, 1843 (1959).
11. R. C. COOKSON and M. E. TREVETT, *J. Chem. Soc.*, 3121 (1956).
12. Z. VALENTA and K. WIESNER, *Chem. and Ind.*, 354 (1956).
13. R. C. COOKSON, J. E. PAGE and M. E. TREVETT, *J. Chem. Soc.*, 4028 (1954).
14. O. E. EDWARDS and L. MARION, *Canad. J. Chem.*, **30**, 627 (1952).
15. O. E. EDWARDS, L. MARION, and D. K. R. STEWART, *Canad. J. Chem.*, **34**, 1315 (1956).
16. R. C. COOKSON and M. E. TREVETT, *Chem. and Ind.*, 276 (1956).
17. O. E. EDWARDS, L. MARION and K. H. PALMER, *J. Org. Chem.*, **22**, 1372 (1957).
18. O. E. EDWARDS and L. MARION, *Canad. J. Chem.*, **32**, 195, 1146 (1954).
19. O. E. EDWARDS and L. MARION, *Canad. J. Chem.*, **30**, 627 (1952).
20. Z. VALENTA and I. G. WRIGHT, *Tetrahedron*, **9**, 284 (1960).
21. O. E. EDWARDS, M. LOSS, and L. MARION, *Proc. Chem. Soc.*, 192 (1959); *Canad. J. Chem.*, **37**, 1996 (1959).
22. R. C. COOKSON and M. E. TREVETT, *J. Chem. Soc.*, 2689, 3864 (1956).
23. M. CARMACK, D. W. MAYE and J. P. FERRIS, *J. Amer. Chem. Soc.*, **80**, 497 (1958); **81**, 4110 (1959).
24. O. E. EDWARDS, L. MARION and K. H. PALMER, *Canad. J. Chem.*, **36**, 1097 (1958).
25. W. I. TAYLOR, W. E. WALLES and L. MARION, *Canad. J. Chem.*, **32**, 780 (1954).
26. E. OCHIAI, T. OKAMOTO, and M. KANEKO, *Chem. and Pharm. Bull.*, **6**, 730 (1958).
27. T. AMIYA and T. SHIMA, *Bull. Chem. Soc. Japan,* **31**, 1083 (1958).
28. H. SUGINOME and S. FURUSAWA, *Bull. Chem. Soc. Japan*, **32**, 354 (1959).
29. S. FURUSAWA, *Bull. Chem. Soc. Japan,* **32**, 399 (1959).
30. V. SKARIC and L. MARION, *J. Amer. Chem. Soc.*, **80**, 4434 (1958); *Canad. J. Chem.*, **38**, 2433 (1960).
31. R. ANET, D. W. CLAYTON and L. MARION, *Canad. J. Chem.*, **35**, 397 (1957).
32. F. SPARATORE, R. GREENHALGH and L. MARION, *Tetrahedron*, **4**, 157 (1958).
33. R. ANET and L. MARION, *Canad. J. Chem.*, **36**, 766 (1958).
34. V. SKARIC and L. MARION, *Canad. J. Chem.*, **39**, 1579 (1961).
35. M. PRZYBYLSKA quoted in ref. 3.
36. M. H. BENN, M. A. M. CAMERON, and O. E. EDWARDS, *Canad. J. Chem.*, **41**, 477 (1963).
37. M. H. BENN, *Canad. J. Chem.*, **44**, 1 (1966).
38. J. B. GROVES, *Pharm. J.*, **8**, 121 (1860).
39. R. MAJIMA, H. SUGINOME, and S. MORIO, *Ber.*, **57**, 1456, 1461, 1472 (1924).
40. R. MAJIMA and S. MORIO, *Annalen*, **476**, 171, 194, 203 (1929).
41. W. A. JACOBS and R. C. ELDERFIELD, *J. Amer. Chem. Soc.*, **58**, 1059 (1936).
42. R. MAJIMA and K. TAMURA, *Annalen*, **526**, 116 (1936).
43. G. H. BECKETT and C. R. WRIGHT, *J. Chem. Soc.*, **29**, 1265 (1875).
44. M. PRZYBYLSKA and L. MARION, *Canad. J. Chem.*, **37**, 1116 (1959).
45. H. MAYER and L. MARION, *Canad. J. Chem.*, **37**, 856 (1959).
46. K. WIESNER, M. GÖTZ, D. L. SIMMONS, L. R. FOWLER, F. W. BACHELOR, R. F. C. BROWN, and G. BUCHI, *Tetrahedron Letters,* No. 2, 15, (1959).
47. F. W. BACHELOR, R. F. C. BROWN and G. BUCHI, *Tetrahedron Letters*, **10**, 1 (1960).
48. L. C. CRAIG, W. A. JACOBS, and R. E. ELDERFIELD, *J. Biol. Chem.*, **128**, 439 (1939).
49. W. A. JACOBS and L. C. CRAIG, *J. Biol. Chem.*, **136**, 323 (1940).
50. W. A. JACOBS and S. W. PELLETIER, *Chem. and Ind.*, 591 (1960).
51. R. B. TURNER, J. P. JESKE and M. S. GIBSON, *J. Amer. Chem. Soc.*, **82**, 5182 (1960).
52. D. J. MCCALDIN and L. MARION, *Canad. J. Chem.*, **37**, 1070 (1959).
53. Y. TSUDA and L. MARION, *Canad. J. Chem.*, **41**, 1485 (1963).
54. K. WIESNER, D. L. SIMMONS and L. R. FOWLER, *Tetrahedron Letters*, No. 8, 1 (1959).

55. C. R. A. WRIGHT and A. P. LUFF, *J. Chem. Soc.*, **33**, 151 (1878).
56. W. R. DUNSTAN and F. H. CARR, *J. Chem. Soc.*, **71**, 350 (1897).
57. T. A. HENRY and T. M. SHARP, *J. Chem. Soc.*, 1105 (1928).
58. T. M. SHARP, *J. Chem. Soc.*, 3094 (1928).
59. W. R. DUNSTAN and A. E. ANDREWS, *J. Chem. Soc.*, **87**, 1620 (1905).
60. R. E. GILMAN and L. MARION, *Canad. J. Chem.*, **42**, 2700 (1964); *Tetrahedron Letters*, 923 (1962).
61. Y. TSUDA and L. MARION, *Canad. J. Chem.*, **41**, 1485 (1963).
62. W. R. DUNSTAN and A. E. ANDREWS, *J. Chem. Soc.*, **87**, 1636 (1905).
63. Y. TSUDA and L. MARION, *Canad. J. Chem.*, **41**, 3055 (1963).
64. O. ACHMATOWICZ and L. MARION, *Canad. J. Chem.*, **42**, 154 (1964).
65. O. ACHMATOWICZ, Y. TSUDA, L. MARION, T. OKAMOTO, M. NATSUME, H. H. CHANG, and K. KOJIMA, *Canad. J. Chem.*, **43**, 825 (1965).
66. O. E. EDWARDS, L. FONZES and L. MARION, *Canad. J. Chem.*, **44**, 583 (1966).
67. S. W. PELLETIER, L. H. KEITH and P. C. PARTHASARATHY, *Tetrahedron Letters*, 4217 (1966).
68. W. A. JACOBS and L. C. CRAIG, *J. Biol. Chem.*, **127**, 361 (1939) *et seq.*
69. W. A. JACOBS and S. W. PELLETIER, *J. Amer. Chem. Soc.*, **78**, 3542 (1956).
70. W. A. JACOBS and S. W. PELLETIER, *J. Amer. Chem. Soc.*, **76**, 161 (1954).
71. W. A. JACOBS and L. C. HUEBNER, *J. Biol. Chem.*, **169**, 211; **170**, 209 (1947).
72. K. WIESNER, F. BICKELHAUPT, D. R. BABIN and M. GÖTZ, *Tetrahedron*, **9**, 254 (1960).
73. W. A. JACOBS and L. C. CRAIG, *J. Biol. Chem.*, **143**, 605 (1942); **147**, 571 (1943).
74. M. PRZYBYLSKA, *Canad. J. Chem.*, **41**, 2911 (1963).
75. R. ANEJA and S. W. PELLETIER, *Tetrahedron Letters*, 669 (1964).
76. O. E. EDWARDS and C. FERRARI, *Canad. J. Chem.*, **42**, 172 (1964).
77. R. ANEJA and S. W. PELLETIER, *Tetrahedron Letters*, 215 (1965).

CHAPTER 7

THE SYNTHESIS OF THE TETRACYCLIC DITERPENES

DURING the past two decades the study of the conformational aspects of reactivity has led to an increasing control over the stereochemical consequences of chemical reactions with widespread ramifications in the synthesis of natural products. Parallel to the early studies on steroid synthesis, work was begun on diterpene synthesis but this did not come to fruition until 1954 when the total synthesis of the aromatic tricyclic diterpene (±)-ferruginol was published.[1] Although this constituted the first synthesis of the racemic form of a naturally occurring diterpene, correctly substituted octahydrophenanthrenes of undefined stereochemistry had been produced by very similar methods in 1939[2] and 1946.[3] The earlier synthesis of di- and triterpenes have been reviewed.[4] For convenience of stereochemical representation, in the sequel the formulae for only one enantiomer are drawn, although in most cases the syntheses have involved racemates. Where possible the naturally occurring enantiomer has been used to enable comparison to be made with the natural product.

7.1. *The Synthesis of Phyllocladene-Kaurene*

The synthesis of the tetracyclic diterpenes fell into a number of stages culminating in the synthesis of the alkaloids. The first stage involved the synthesis of intermediates in which ring C remained aromatic. The majority of the syntheses of tricyclic intermediates of this type had as their goal compounds of the diterpenoid resin acid series. However, experience in this area led to control over two major stereochemical features of the tetracyclic series—the geminal substituents at C-4 and the A/B fusion. In the second stage ring C was reduced and the corresponding perhydrophenanthrenes alkylated at C-8. Here the angular methyl group exerted a control over the incoming group and thus direct alkylation led to a residue at C-8 *trans* to the C-10 angular methyl group (i.e. with the kaurene B/C fusion). The final stages in the formation of ring D were remarkable for the ease with which cyclization reactions occur between C-8 and C-13 residues.

The first stage involved routes which drew heavily on experience obtained in the steroid field. Although it is analogous to part of the proposed biogenetic route to the diterpenes, the use of acid-catalysed multiple cyclizations of either completely aliphatic systems, or ω-phenyl alkenols[5,8] affords little control over the stereochemistry of the resultant ring junctions. The use of epoxides seems to afford more promise. The routes used in building up the tricyclic system involved either the construction of rings A and C and their subsequent cyclization to form ring B or the use of a ring extension reaction to add ring A to a tetralone which contained the features of rings B and C. Thus the ethers (I) and (II) were synthesized[9–11] and used as intermediates in the synthesis of di- and tricyclic diterpenes.

The first method was exemplified[9] by the condensation of *m*-methoxyphenyl acetylene and 2, 2, 6-trimethylcyclohexanone. Reduction of the ethynylcarbinol and cyclization with polyphosphoric acid gave the tricyclic ether (I). Cyclizations of this type led to separable mixtures of *cis* and *trans* fused isomers. In this particular instance the presence of a methoxyl group *para* to the newly formed bond permitted thermodynamic control of the cyclization and thus the predominance of the *trans* isomer. A novel route to the tricyclic ether (I) used[10] the base-catalysed condensation of *m*-methoxybenzaldehyde with isopropyl methyl ketone. The resultant unsaturated ketone (III) was then condensed with the Mannich base, 1-diethylamino-3-pentanone methiodide, to form a dienone which on subsequent reduction and cyclization gave the tricyclic ether (I). In the cases bearing a carboxyl substituent at C-4 further isomerism was possible. In the event all four isomers of desoxypodocarpic acid were isolated and their relative configurations assigned.[12]

Syntheses utilizing a tetralone intermediate afforded a greater control over both A/B fusion and the stereochemistry at C-4, as exemplified[13] by the synthesis of (±)-dehydroabietic acid. Thus ring extension of the tetralone (IV) with ethylvinyl ketone gave the tricyclic ketone (V). The angular methyl directed alkylation with bromoacetic ester and hydrogenation to occur from the less-hindered opposite face of the molecule. Further manipulation then led to (±)-dehydroabietic acid(VI). Another example of this approach is found in the total synthesis of (±)-kaur-16-en-19-oic acid (*vide infra*).

In the second stage of the syntheses the aromatic ring C was reduced and the corresponding perhydrophenanthrene ketones alkylated at C-8. Since the angular methyl groups at C-10 directs *trans* alkylation at C-8 it was necessary in the synthesis of the degradation product (IX) of phyllocladene in which the carbomethoxyl group represented the residue of ring D, to cleave ring C after alkylation and reclose the ring by a base-catalysed condensation to form the more stable trans-*anti*-trans backbone of phyllocladene.

Thus the α-methylene position of the ketone (VII) was blocked[11] as its furfurylidene derivative and the ketone then alkylated with allyl

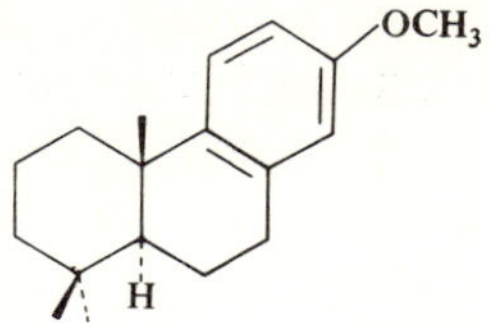

OCH_3 H

I

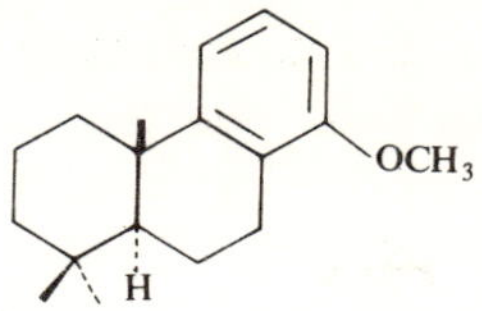

OCH_3 H

II

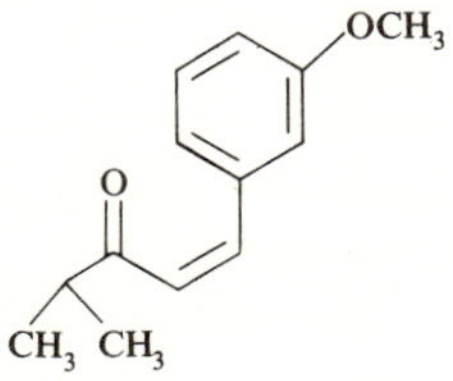

OCH_3 O CH_3 CH_3

III

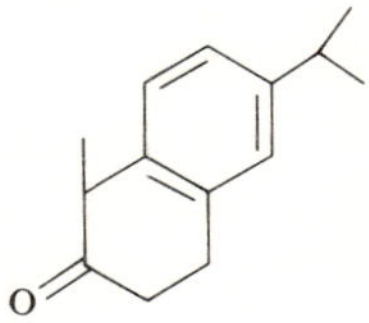

O

IV

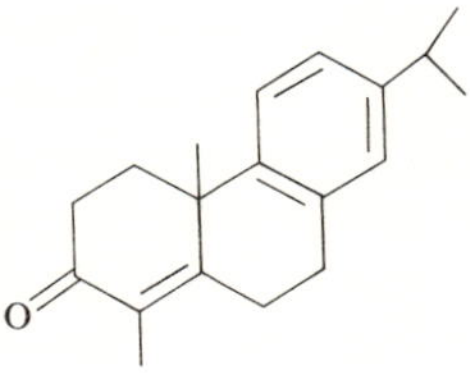

O

V

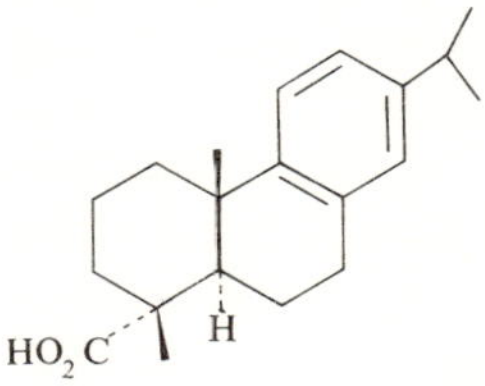

HO_2C H

VI

bromide. Ozonolysis and esterification gave the tri-ester (VIII) which underwent Dieckmann cyclization to form the keto-ester (IX). This degradation product of phyllocladene was also synthesized[10] from the unsaturated ketone, $\Delta^{8,14}$-podocarpen-7-one (X), a compound which had been a fruitful intermediate[14,15] for syntheses of bi- and tricyclic diterpenoids. Reduction of the unsaturated ketone gave the epimeric allylic alcohols. The predominant equatorial isomer gave a vinyl ether which on Claisen rearrangement and oxidation gave an acid (XI). This acid on ozonolysis and partial methylation gave an anhydride ester which underwent a similar Dieckmann cyclization to the keto-ester (IX).

A total synthesis[16] of methyl (±)-8α-carboxymethylpodocarpan-13-one-4β-carboxylate (XII) which is a degradation product of steviol followed a similar pattern. The tricyclic $\alpha\beta$-unsaturated keto-ester (XIII)[17] was reduced to an allylic alcohol and the corresponding vinyl ether rearranged and oxidized to form an unsaturated acid analogous to (XI). Hydroxylation of the $\Delta^{7,8}$ double bonded to a γ-lactone in turn oxidized to an α-keto-lactone. On hydrogenolysis and methylation this gave the required keto-ester.

The synthesis of phyllocladene was completed by a Reformatsky

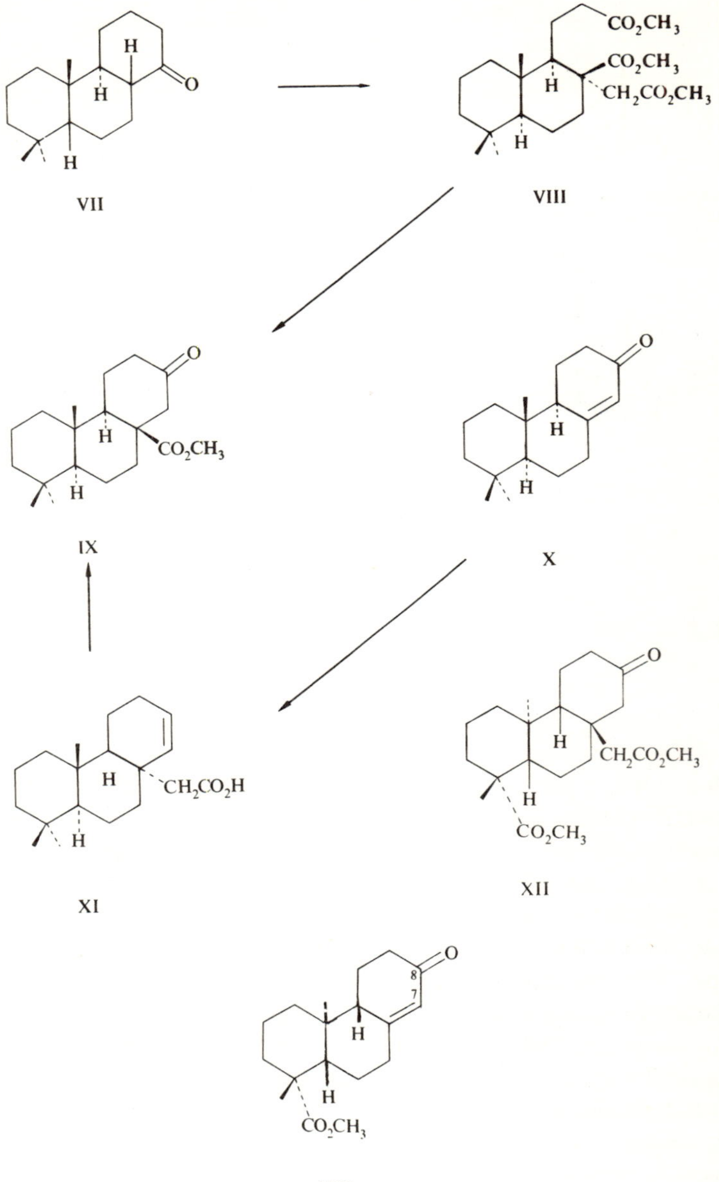
VII
VIII
IX
X
XI
XII
XIII
CO2CH3
CH2CO2CH3
CH2CO2H

reaction on the keto-ester (XIV) forming the γ-lactone (XV) which was in turn converted through a saturated dicarboxylic acid to the cyclopentanone (XVI) and thence to (±)-phyllocladene (XVII).

The total synthesis of (±)-kaurene (XXI) on the other hand was completed[19] by hydroboronation of the ethylene acetal of the unsaturated

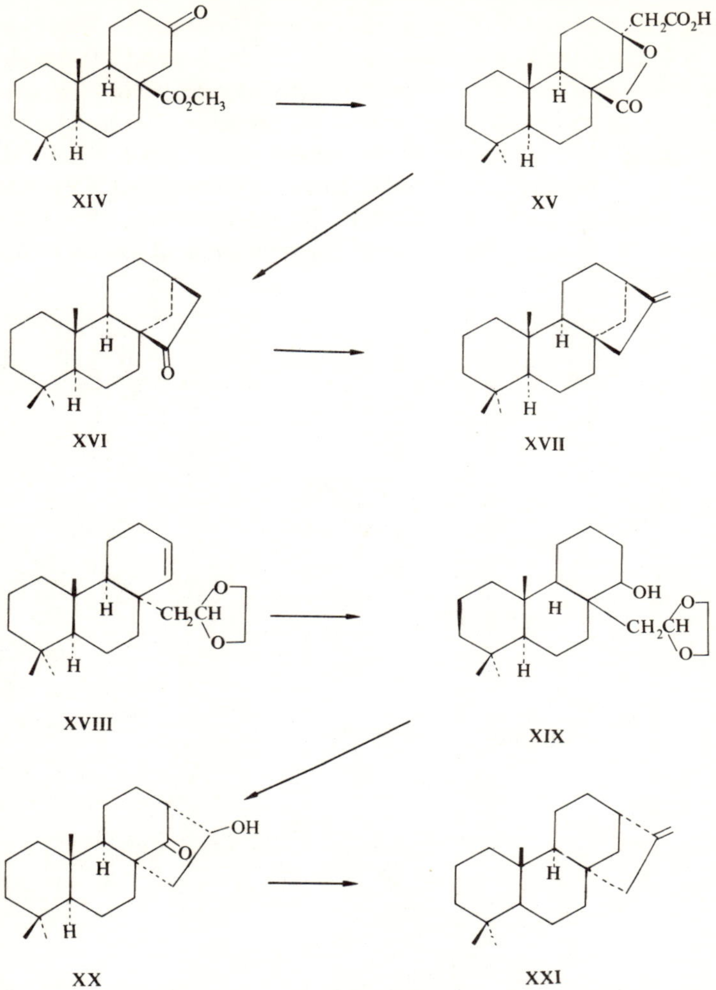

XIV

XV

XVI

XVII

XVIII

XIX

XX

XXI

aldehyde (XVIII) related to the acid (XI) used in the cleavage of ring C mentioned above. One of the products was the hydroxy-acetal (XIX) which was readily converted through oxidation hydrolysis and internal aldol condensation to the tetracyclic hydroxy-ketone (XX). Several subsequent stages led to (±)-kaurene (XXI). The 14-ketone was considerably more hindered than the 16-ketone and thus even in the presence of excess methylenephosphorane, the diketone gave (±)-14-ketokaurene which was subsequently reduced to (±)-kaurene (XXI).

A variant on this method was employed[20] in the synthesis of (±)-kaur-16-en-19-oic acid (XXVI)—the first synthesis of a compound with gibberellin-like activity. The tetralone, 1-methyl-5-methoxy-tetrahydronaphthalen-2-one, was condensed with methyl acroylacetate. Methylation and stepwise reduction of resultant tricyclic keto-ester (XXII) gave the ester (XXIII). Ring D was then constructed by Ireland's method. That is C-7 was blocked with the n-butyl thiomethylene protecting group and the angular position alkylated with allyl bromide. Removal of the protecting group and cleavage of the double bond gave a keto-aldehyde (XXIV) which readily condensed to a hydroxy-ketone (XXV). Reduction of the 14-ketone and oxidation of the 16-hydroxyl afforded (±)-17-norkauran-19-oic acid from which the parent acid (XXVI) had been reconstituted.

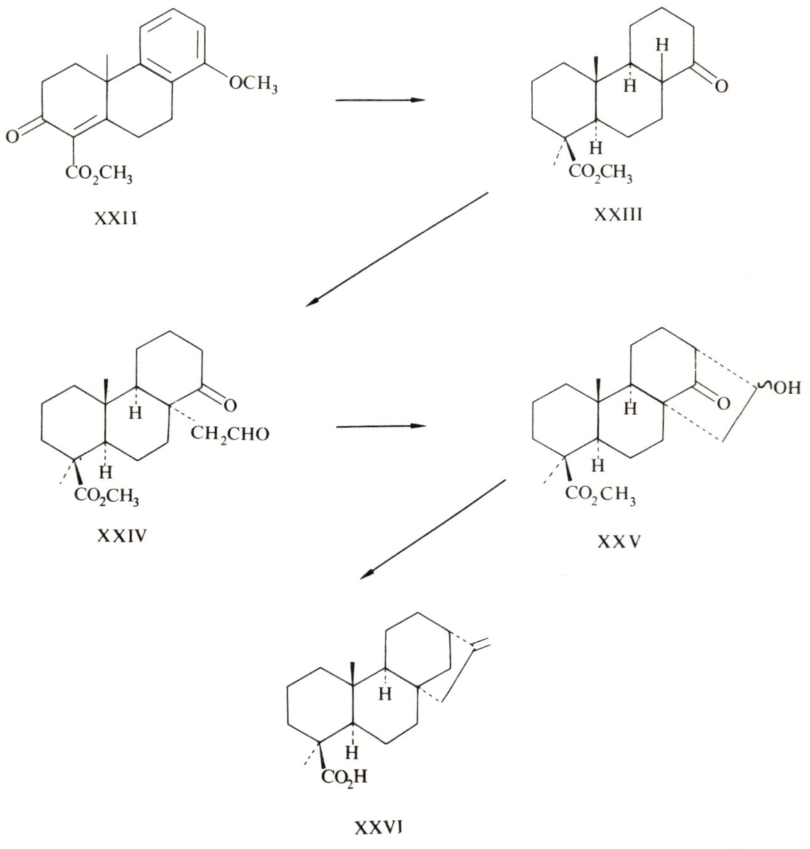

XXII

XXIII

XXIV

XXV

XXVI

The keto-acetal (XXVII) formed the basis of a synthesis[2] of (±)-hibaene (XXXI). Conversion to the methyl ketone (XXVIII) was followed by cyclization to the tetracyclic system (XXIX) possessing the kauranoid stereochemistry. Beckmann rearrangement of the oximinoacetate led to the introduction of a bridgehead function. Further transformation gave a hydroxyolefin (XXX) analogous to steviol which underwent a Wagner–Meerwein rearrangement to a ketone with the hibaene skeleton. The total

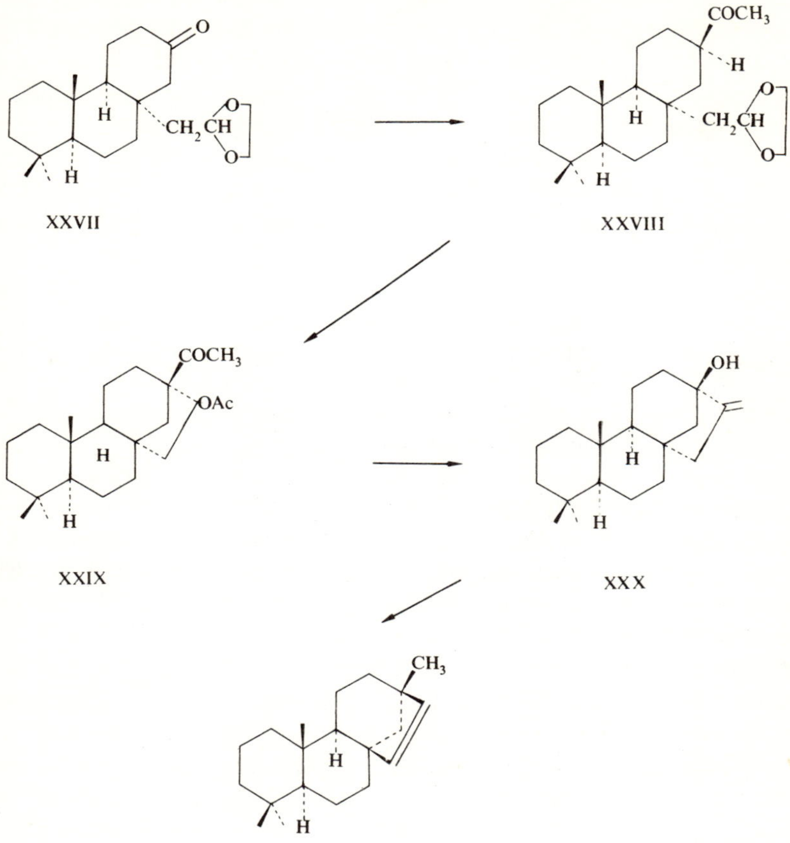

XXVII

XXVIII

XXIX

XXX

XXXI

synthesis of (±)-hibaene (XXXI) was then completed when this ketone was reduced with sodium borohydride and the Δ^{15}-olefinic bond introduced through elimination of the derived tosylate.

An elegant synthesis of kaurene, the Garrya alkaloids and the atisine alkaloids has been reported[22] in which the tetracyclic keto-acid (XXXII) forms a key tetracyclic common intermediate. This intermediate could be obtained by degradation of veatchine. Reduction of the angular substituent to a methyl group led to kaurene norketone. Alternatively conversion to the azide and subsequent photolysis permitted the construction of the heterocyclic ring of the alkaloids and hence to a partial synthesis of garryine. Alternatively the ring D intermediate (XXXIII) involved in the garryine synthesis was degraded to a keto-ester (XXXIV) and the latter carboxymethylated and reduced to a tricyclic ester related to atisine.

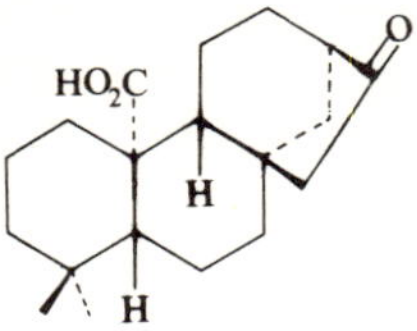

HO_2C H H O

XXXII

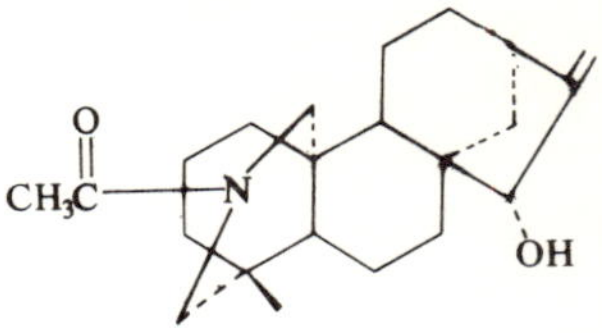

CH_3C O N OH

XXXIII

CO_2CH_3 CH_3CO N CO_2CH_3

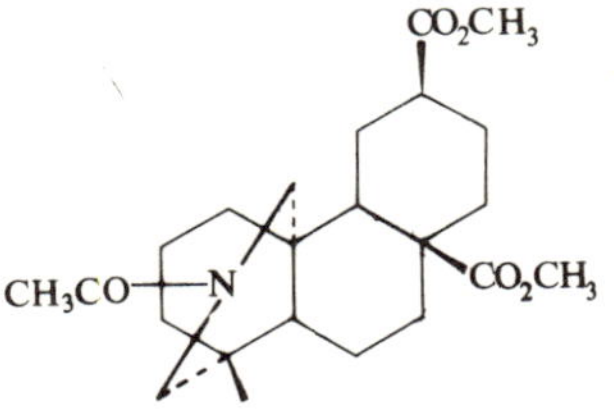

XXXIV

7.2. *The Synthesis of the Alkaloids*

Considerable effort has been directed at the total synthesis of the alkaloids, which involves not only the porblem of constructing the carbon skeleton but also that of the heterocyclic rings E and F. A number of solutions to this problem have been published recently.

A stereospecific synthesis of DL-atisine involved[23] construction of the heterocyclic ring first. Thus addition of hydrogen cyanide to the unsaturated ketone (XXXV) gave the angular nitrile (XXXVI) in turn converted by a Wittig reaction to the aldehyde and then methylated. Transannular cyclization led to the formation of an amide which was reduced with lithium aluminium hydride to cyclic amine. Alternatively, reduction of the nitrile led to a primary amino alcohol whose dimesyl derivative underwent cyclization. Birch reduction of ring C and rearrangement of the resulting enol ether gave the podocarpenone (XXXVII). Elaboration of ring D of atisine then followed the sequence (XXXVIII) to (XLIV). Of particular interest in this work is the cleavage of ring D by elimination of the mesylate. The reconstruction of the six-membered ring D of atisine followed by utilizing hydroboronation of the olefin in (XL) and internal alkylation of

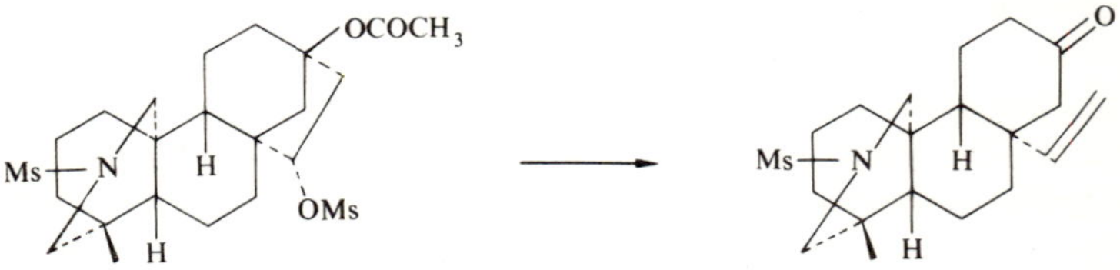

$OCOCH_3$ Ms N H OMs H → Ms N H H O

XXXIX XL

ring C. The formation of the allylic alcohol system involved an unusual pathway. Bromination of (XLIII) gave the Δ^{15}-allylic bromide which on epoxydation reputedly gave the 15β-epoxide. This was reduced with zinc and ethanol to the β-allylic alcohol. Comparison with reactions in the kaurene series would suggest the opposite stereochemistry. A variation on this route provided[23] a synthesis of the Garrya alkaloids. It involved an interesting rearrangement of rings C and D. In the olefin (XLV) the heterocyclic ring and double bond are on the same side of the molecule.

XXXV

XXXVI

XXXVII

XXXVIII

XXXIX

XL

XLI

XLII

XLIII

XLIV

Hydroboronation gave the exocyclic alcohol (XLVI). Treatment of the brosylate with aqueous potassium hydroxide smoothly gave the ketone (XLVII) possessing the kauranoid stereochemistry. Elaboration of the allylic alcohol followed the atisine synthesis.

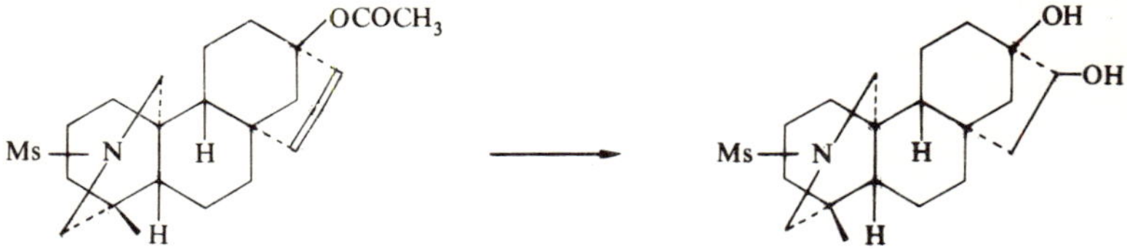

XLV

XLVI

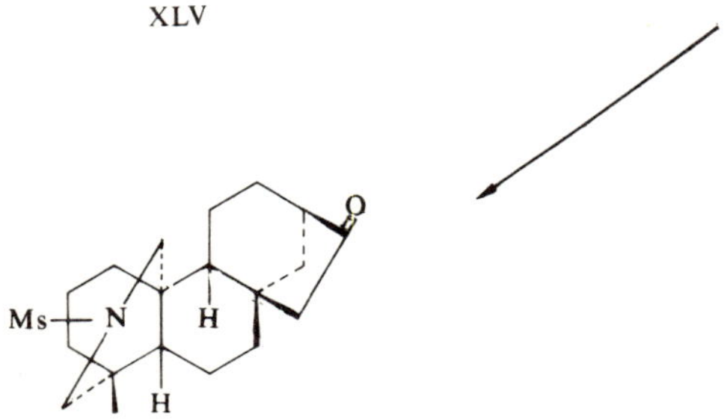

XLVII

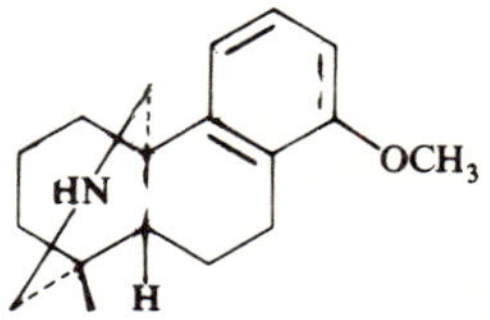

XLVIII

Another synthesis of the Garrya alkaloids followed closely the synthetic route to (±)-kaur-16-en-19-oic acid[20] and (±)-kaurene[19] described earlier. In this synthesis the key intermediate amine (XLVIII) was prepared[24,25] by a number of routes. The subsequent elaboration of ring D by reduction[26] of the aromatic ring and alkylation followed the earlier work. Several other syntheses of fragments of the carbon skeleton have been briefly described.[27,31] A partial synthesis of the atisine skeleton from abietic acid derivatives has led to compounds with the enantiomeric absolute stereochemistry.[32]

7.3. *The Synthesis of the Gibberellins*

A number of approaches have been made in the synthesis of suitably substituted hexahydrofluorenes related[33–36] to degradation products of gibberellic acid. Cyclization of 1-cyclohexenylphenyl and 1-cyclohexenyl *o*-tolyl ketones with polyphosphoric acid as model systems gave predominantly the *cis*-hexahydrofluorenones. However, the stereochemistry of the products of cyclization of trans-2-phenylcyclohexanol with aluminium trichloride was dependent on the catalyst ratio.

The synthesis of gibberone was achieved[37–39] through the unsaturated keto-acid (L) prepared by reacting the enol of t-butyl-4-methyl-1-oxoindan-2-yl acetic acid (XLIX) with isopropenyl methyl ketone. Internal electrophilic acylation led to the cyclization of this acid to a diketone which on selective reduction gave (±)-gibberone (LI). The intermediate acid has also been prepared[39] independently from 4-methylindan-2-one through the spiro-diketone (LII). An extension of this synthesis led to[40] (±)-gibberic acid (LIII).

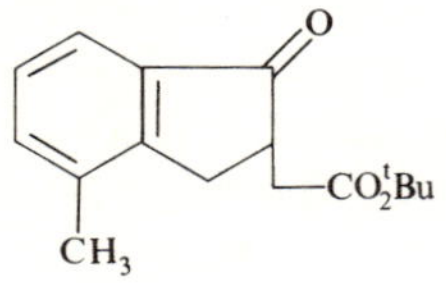

XLIX

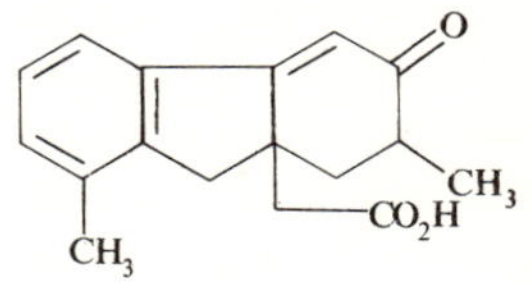

L

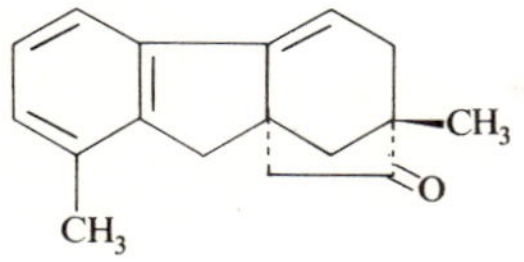

LI

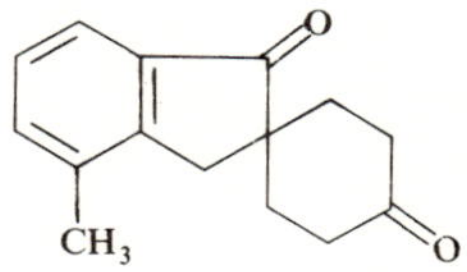

LII

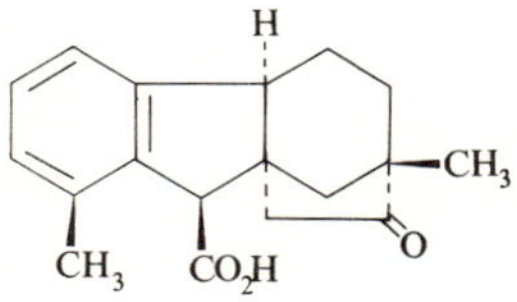

LIII

The Japanese group of workers have been extremely active in the synthesis of compounds related to the gibberellins. The stages in this work have involved first the synthesis of gibberone, then gibberic acid, followed by the reconstitution of ring A. Two reaction schemes have been explored, both starting from 4-methylhydrindanone. Initially 7-demethyldihydrogibberone was obtained[41] as follows. Alkylation of 2-carbomethoxy-4-methylhydrindone with methyl bromoacetate followed by acid-hydrolysis gave the acid (LIV). This was subjected to a Robinson ring extension reaction to form the tetrahydrofluorenone (LV) from which (±)-7-demethyl-6-ketogibberone (LVI) was obtained by refluxing the acid with boron trifluoride etherate in glacial acetic acid. Selective ketalization followed by reduction and hydrolysis of the ketal gave 7-demethylgibberone. Hydrogenation, assumed to take place from the α-face of the molecule, then gave 7-demethyldihydrogibberone—a degradation product of gibberellins A_9 and A_{13}.

An extension of this approach led to the total synthesis of (±)-epigibberic acid and (±)-gibberic acid. Thus annelation of the hydrinanone[42] (LVII) with isopropenyl methyl ketone afforded the fluorenone (LVIII).[43] The relative configuration of the carboxyl was fixed by their conversion to a *cis* anhydride. Treatment of this anhydride with boron trifluoride etherate in acetic acid afforded a diketo-acid. The steric course of hydrogenation of the $\Delta^{4b:5}$ double bond is determined by the orientation of the 10-carboxyl group. Thus hydrogenation of the monoketal of (LIX) followed by appropriate modification of the functional groups including epimerization of the ester afforded (±)-epigibberic acid (LX). Alternatively, epimerization of the ester grouping prior to reduction led via (±)-dehydrogibberic acid to (±)-gibberic acid (LIII). A number of desoxy relatives were also prepared.[44]

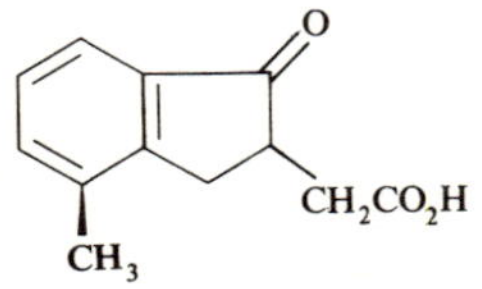

O
CH_2CO_2H
CH_3

LIV

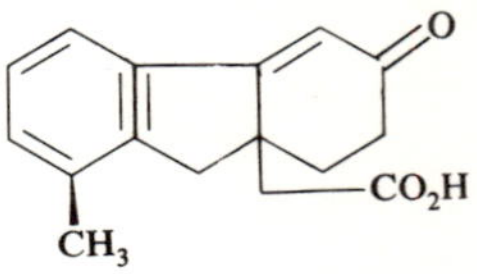

O
CO_2H
CH_3

LV

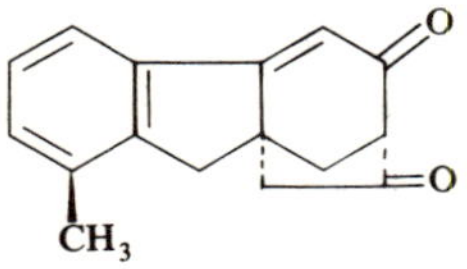

O
O
CH_3

LVI

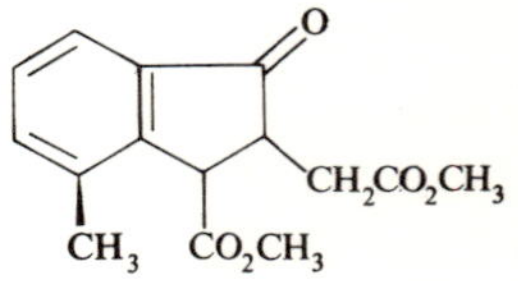

O
$CH_2CO_2CH_3$
CH_3 CO_2CH_3

LVII

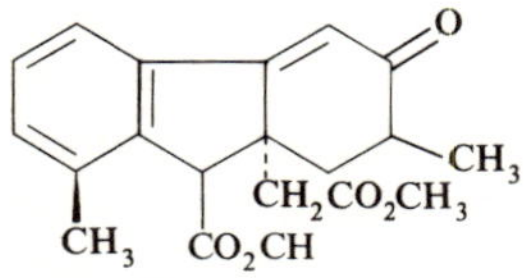

O
CH_3
$CH_2CO_2CH_3$
CH_3 CO_2CH

LVIII

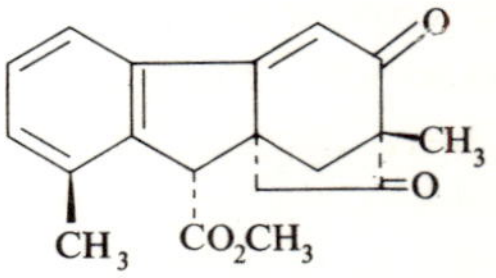

O
CH_3
O
CH_3 CO_2CH_3

LIX

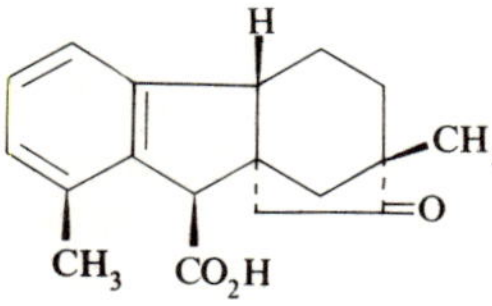

H
CH_3
O
CH_3 CO_2H

LX

An alternative scheme developed by the same group of workers utilized the Diels–Alder reaction between the ketal (LXI) and butadiene. The ketone (LXII) corresponding to the adduct was then converted by a ring-extension reaction to the tetracyclic ketone (LXIII). Cleavage of the olefin and cyclization of the resultant dicarboxylic acid led[45] to a compound in the 6-keto dehydrohomogibberic acid series (LXIV).

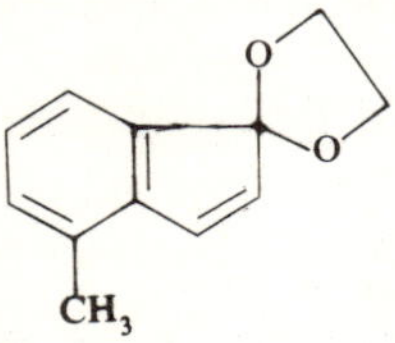

CH_3

LXI

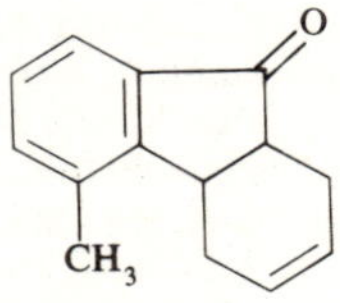

CH_3

LXII

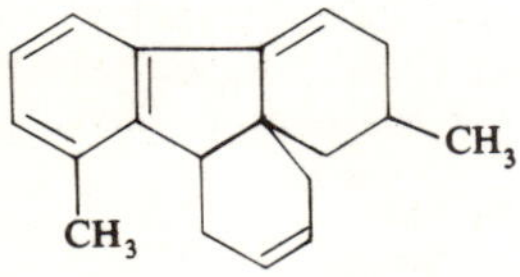

CH_3 CH_3

LXIII

CH_3 CH_3 CH_2CO_2H O

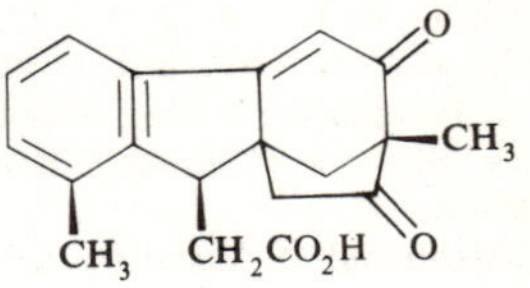

LXIV

Some progress has been made in the synthesis of ring A of the gibberellins although in very low yield. Thus the saturated ring A of (LXVI) has been reconstructed from the dienone (LXV) by carbonation followed by relactonization. Another approach[47] is exemplified by reduction of the aromatic acid (LXVII) with sodium in liquid ammonia and methylation

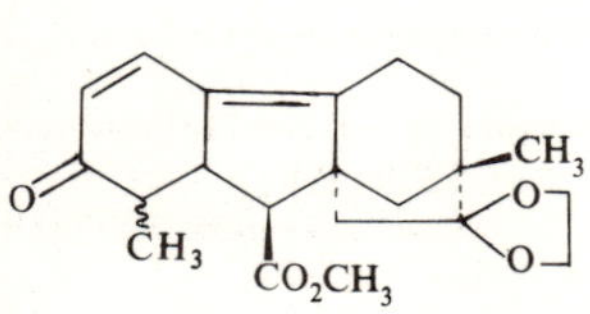

CH_3 CH_3 CO_2CH_3

LXV

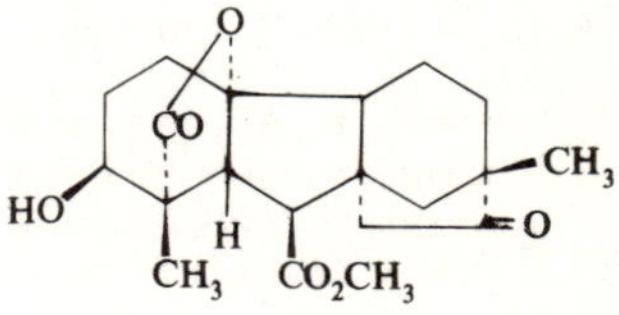

HO CO H CH_3 CH_3 CO_2CH_3 O

LXVI

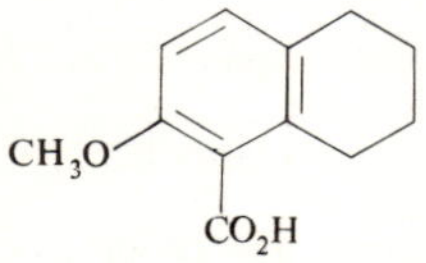

CH_3O CO_2H

LXVII

O CO H

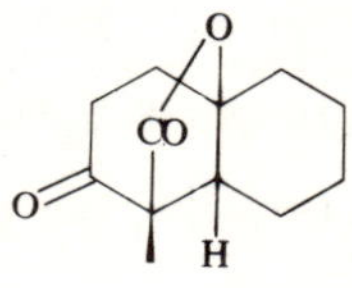

LXVIII

of the carbanion with methyl iodide. Relactonization led to the keto-lactone (LXVIII).

REFERENCES

1. F. G. King, T. J. King, and J. G. Topliss, *Chem. and Ind.*, 108 (1954); *J. Chem. Soc.*, 573 (1957).
2. R. D. Haworth and R. L. Barker, *J. Chem. Soc.*, 1299 (1939).
3. R. D. Haworth and B. P. Moore, *J. Chem. Soc.*, 633 (1946); B. K. Bhattacharya, *J. Ind. Chem. Soc.*, **22**, 165 (1945).
4. N. A. J. Rogers and J. A. Barltrop, *Quart. Rev.*, **16**, 117 (1962).
5. M. Fetizon, *Compt. Rend.*, **246**, 2774 (1958).
6. D. Nasipuri, *Chem. and Ind.*, 424 (1957).
7. M. F. Ansell and A. Selleck, *J. Chem. Soc.*, 1238 (1956).
8. A. Caliezi and H. Schinz, *Helv. Chim. Acta*, **35**, 1649 (1952).
9. J. A. Barltrop and N. A. J. Rogers, *Chem. and Ind.*, 20 (1957); *J. Chem. Soc.*, 2546 (1958).
10. R. F. Church, R. E. Ireland, and J. A. Marshall, *Tetrahedron Letters*, No. 17, 1 (1960).
11. R. B. Turner and P. E. Shaw, *Tetrahedron Letters*, No. 18, 24 (1960).
12. U. R. Ghatak, *Tetrahedron Letters*, No. 1, 19 (1959); U. R. Ghatak, P. C. Datta and J. R. Ray, *J. Amer. Chem. Soc.*, **82**, 1728 (1960).
13. G. Stork and J. W. Schulenberg, *J. Amer. Chem. Soc.*, **78**, 250 (1956).
14. J. A. Barltrop, N. A. J. Rogers and D. B. Bigley, *J. Chem. Soc.*, 4613 (1960).
15. J. A. Barltrop, N. A. J. Rogers, D. Giles and J. R. Hanson, *J. Chem. Soc.*, 2534 (1962).
16. K. Mori and M. Matsui, *Tetrahedron Letters*, 2347 (1965).
17. J. A. Barltrop and A. C. Day, *J. Chem. Soc.*, 671 (1959).
18. R. B. Turner and K. H. Ganshirt, *Tetrahedron Letters*, 231 (1961).
19. R. A. Bell, R. E. Ireland, and R. A. Partyka, *J. Org. Chem.*, **27**, 3741 (1962).
20. K. Mori and M. Matsui, *Tetrahedtron Letters*, 175 (1966); K. Mori and M. Matsui, *Tetrahedron*, **24**, 3095 (1968).
21. R. E. Ireland and L. N. Mander, *Tetrahedron Letters*, 2627 (1965).
22. S. Masamune, *J. Amer. Chem. Soc.*, **83**, 1009 (1961); **86**, 288 (1964).
23. W. Nagata, T. Sugasawa, N. Narusada, T. Wakabayashi, Y. Hayase, *J. Amer. Chem. Soc.*, **85**, 2342 (1963); W. Nagata, N. Narisada, T. Wakabayashi, and T. Sugasawa, *J. Amer. Chem. Soc.*, **86**, 929 (1964).
24. J. A. Findlay, W. A. Henry, T. C. Jain, Z. Valenta, K. Wiesner, and C. W. Wong, *Tetrahedron Letters*, 869 (1962).
25. R. W. Guthrie, A. Phillip, Z. Valenta and K. Wiesner, *Tetrahedron Letters*, 2945 (1965).
26. Z. Valenta, K. Wiesner, and C. W. Wong, *Tetrahedron Letters*, 2437 (1964).
27. A. A. Othman and N. A. J. Rogers, *Tetrahedron Letters*, 1339 (1963).
28. W. A. Ayer, C. E. McDonald and G. G. Iverach, *Tetrahedron Letters*, 1095 (1963).
29. O. E. Edwards and J. ApSimon, *Canad. J. Chem.*, **40**, 896 (1962).
30. I. Iwai, A. Ogiso and B. Shimizu, *Chem. and Ind.*, 1288 (1962).
31. S. W. Pelletier and P. C. Pharthasarathy, *Tetrahedron Letters*, 205 (1963).
32. L. H. Zalkow and N. N. Girotra, *J. Org. Chem.*, **28**, 2037 (1963); **29**, 1299 (1964).
33. H. O. House, V. Paragamian, R. S. Ro, and D. J. Wluka, *J. Amer. Chem. Soc.*, **82**, 1452, 1457 (1960).
34. H. O. House, W. F. Gannon, R. S. Ro, and D. J. Wluka, *J. Amer. Chem. Soc.*, **82**, 1463.
35. H. O. House, V. Paragamian and D. J. Wluka, *J. Amer. Chem. Soc.*, **82**, 2561, 2714, (1960).
36. H. O. House, R. G. Carlson, H. Muller, A. W. Noltes, and G. D. Slater, *J. Amer. Chem. Soc.*, **84**, 2614 (1962).
37. H. J. E. Loewenthal, *Proc. Chem. Soc.*, 305 (1960).

38. Y. Nos and H. J. E. Loewenthal, *J. Chem. Soc.*, 605 (1963).
39. T. Money, R. A. Raphael, A. I. Scott and D. W. Young, *J. Chem. Soc.*, 3958 (1961).
40. H. J. E. Loewenthal and S. K. Malhotra, *Proc. Chem. Soc.*, 230 (1962); *J. Chem. Soc.*, 990 (1965).
41. K. Mori, M. Matsui and Y. Sumiki, *Agr. Biol. Chem.*, **25**, 907 (1961).
42. K. Mori, M. Matsui, and Y. Sumiki, *Agr. Biol. Chem.*, **27**, 27 (1963).
43. K. Mori, M. Matsui, and Y. Sumiki, *Agr. Biol. Chem.*, **26**, 783 (1962); **27**, 537 (1963).
44. K. Mori, T. Ogawa, M. Matsui, and Y. Sumiki, *Agr. Biol. Chem.*, **28**, 239 (1964).
45. K. Mori, M. Matsui, and Y. Sumiki, *Agr. Biol. Chem.*, **27**, 22 (1963).
46. K. Mori, M. Matsui, and Y. Sumiki, *Tetrahedron Letters*, 1803 (1964).
47. M. D. Bachi, J. W. Epstein and H. J. E. Loewenthal, *Tetrahedron Letters*, 5333 (1966).

CHAPTER 8

THE BIOSYNTHESIS OF THE TETRACYCLIC DITERPENES

THE tetracyclic diterpenes have provided a fruitful field for biogenetic speculation. The tetracyclic skeleta are sufficiently closely related to suggest a common biosynthetic pathway. A number of schemes have been proposed[1–9] for this pathway. These have to accommodate a number of features. Firstly, in contradistinction to the triterpenes and steroids, a large number of these compounds lack a C-3 oxygen function. Secondly, the antipodal A/B fusion is widespread, almost predominant. Thirdly, there invariably exists a *trans* relationship between the C-10 angular substituent and the 9-hydrogen atom. Fourthly, there exist both bicyclo-3,2,2-octane and several bicyclo-3,2,1-octane systems for rings C and D. Finally, the scheme must account for modification of the perhydrophenanthrene backbone to the perhydrofluorene and perhydrobenzazulene skeleta of the gibberellins and grayanotoxins.

In 1955 Wenkert suggested[2] that the tetracyclic diterpenes might arise through cyclization of suitably oriented pimaradienes (I) involving a non-classical carbonium ion. This ion (II) might collapse in a number of ways forming compounds of the kaurene skeleta (III) the atisine skeleta (IV) and the stachene group (V). Alternatively, cyclization of this ion may lead to the recently discovered penta-cyclic trachylobane skeleton. The co-occurrence[9] of a progenitor of this type, (−)-pimaradiene, with its products of cyclization of (−)-hibaene, and atisirine in *Erythroxylon monogynum* lends valuable support to a theory of this type. With a cyclization of this kind, the C-13 isopimaradienes (VI) could well be the precursor of phyllocladene and the hitherto hypothetical 8,13-isohibaene. Indeed a laboratory analogy[4] in the cyclization of (VII) derived from isopimaric acid to the 8,13-isohibaene ketol (VIII) already exists although this employs base-catalysed conditions. The acid-catalysed cyclization of manool to $\Delta^{8,9}$ isopimaradiene, $\Delta^{8,9}$ sandaracopimaradiene, the rosadienes and hibaene has recently been described.[26] As yet a correlation does not appear to exist between the co-occurrence of bi-, tri- and tetracyclic with a consistent C-13 configuration.

The transformation of the perhydrophenanthrene skeleton of (−)-kaurene to the various rearranged skeleton follows pathways for which

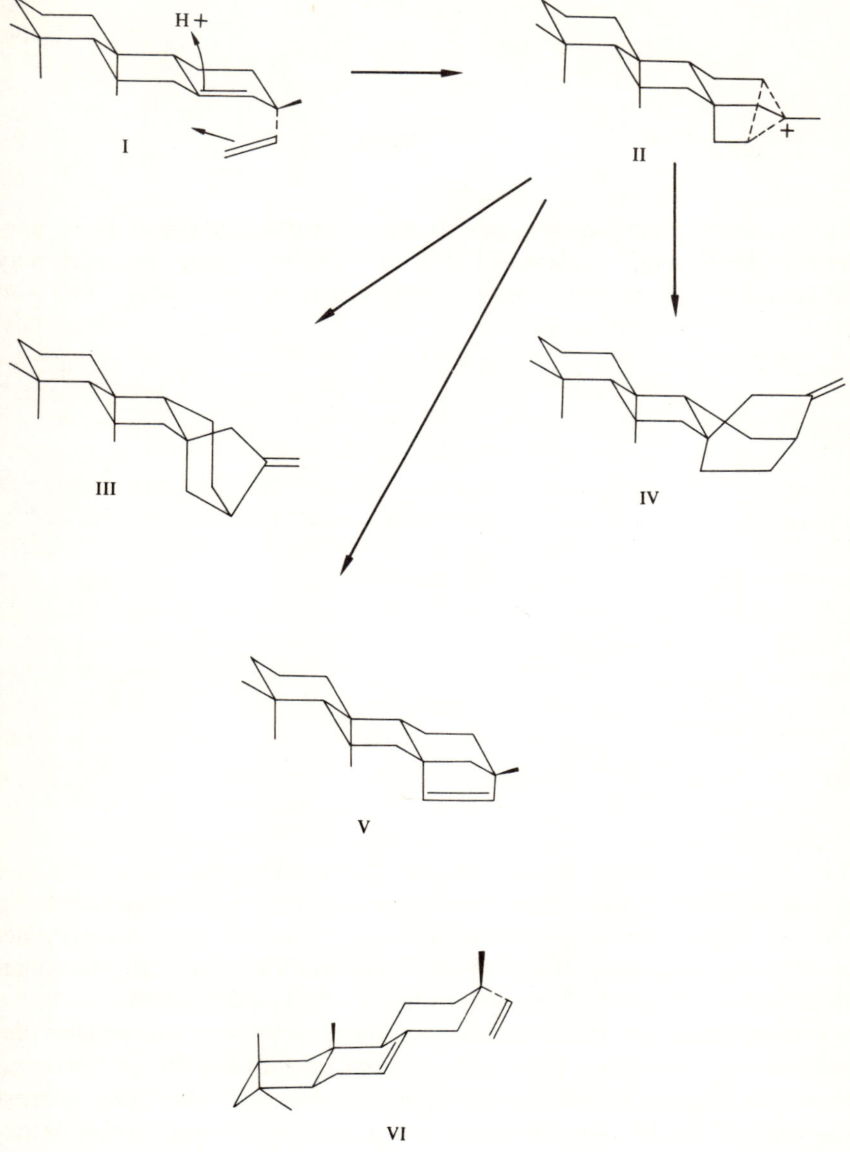

in vitro analogies exist. This has been substantiated[10] in the conversion of (—)-kaurene to gibberellic acid by *G. fujikuroi*. Thus the gibbane skeleton (IX) might arise by migration of the 7,8-bond and extrusion of C-7. Alternatively, migration of the 5, 10-bond to C-1 may lead to the grayanotoxin skeleton (X). The isolation[11] of kauranoid derivatives bearing an equatorial substituent at C-1 is of considerable interest in ths connection.

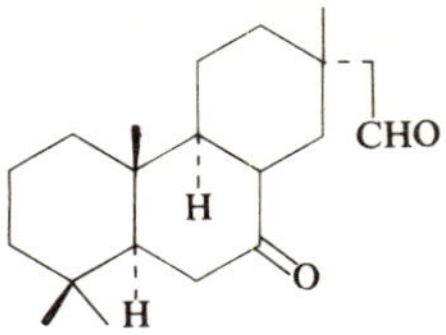

VII

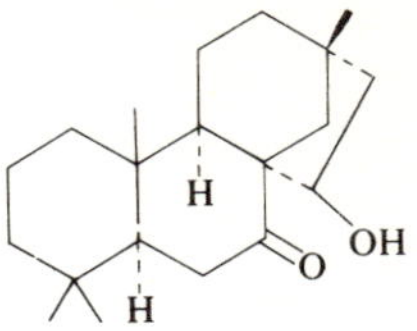

VIII

Furthermore, a simple Wagner–Meerwein rearrangement at C-18 may lead to the furanoid skeleton of cafestol (XI), an analogy to which may be found in the rearrangements at this centre in the abietic[12] and vin-

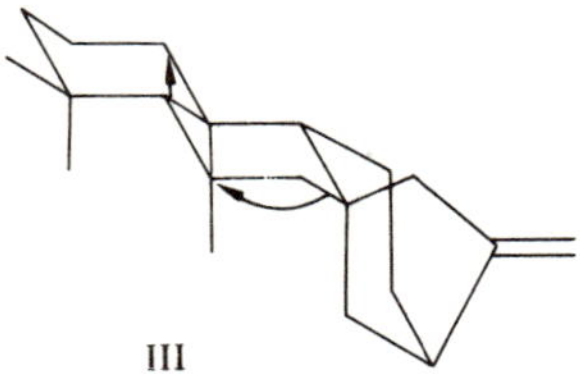

III

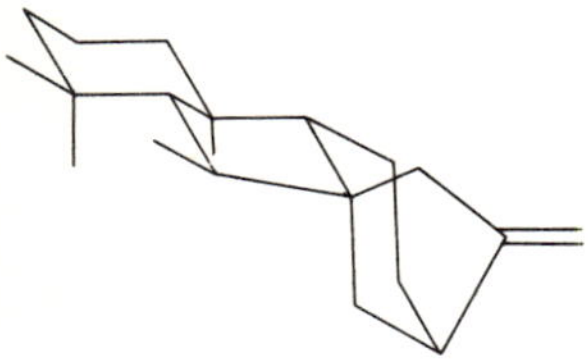

IX

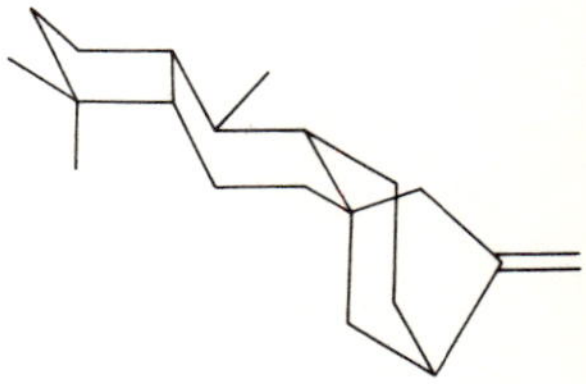

X

haticoic acid[13] series. Cleavage of ring B of (−)-kaurene (XIII) may lead to fujenal (XIV)[14] and thence by rotation about the 9–10 bond to enmein (XV).[15] It has been suggested[16] that the C-19 aconitines (XVII) are derived from compounds of the atisine skeleton (XVI), through rearrangement of the 8,9-bond to 8, 15 and the loss of the 17-substituent.

Experimental evidence to support these schemes is gradually accumulating. Fortunately both the kauranoid and gibbane skeleta are found in the metabolites of the mould, *Gibberella fujikuroi*. Particular interest has centred on the biosynthesis of the gibberellins owing to their widespread effect on higher plants. The biosynthesis of gibberellic acid involves a number of modifications of the tetracyclic precursor. These entail oxidation at C-19, contraction of ring B to form a cyclopentane carboxylic acid, loss of the angular methyl group and lactonization, followed by oxidative modification of ring A and the C/D bridgehead position.

Evidence to support this came from a series of incorporation experiments. Degradation of gibberellic acid isolated[6] from a fermentation to which sodium (1-^{14}C)-acetate had been added, showed radioactivity at the sites marked in (XVIII). This labelling pattern indicated that formation of the tetracyclic skeleton from a tricyclic (—)-pimaradiene precursor required migration of the pimarane C-8–C-18, i.e. it demonstrated that C-8 is involved in the non-classical carbonium ion (II). Four molecules of both (2-^{14}C)- and (4-^{14}C)-mevalonolactone were incorporated into gibberellic acid (XIX; 2-^{14}C = X; 4-^{14}C = •) demonstrating its diterpenoid nature. Two of the labelled atoms were accounted for by the 1-

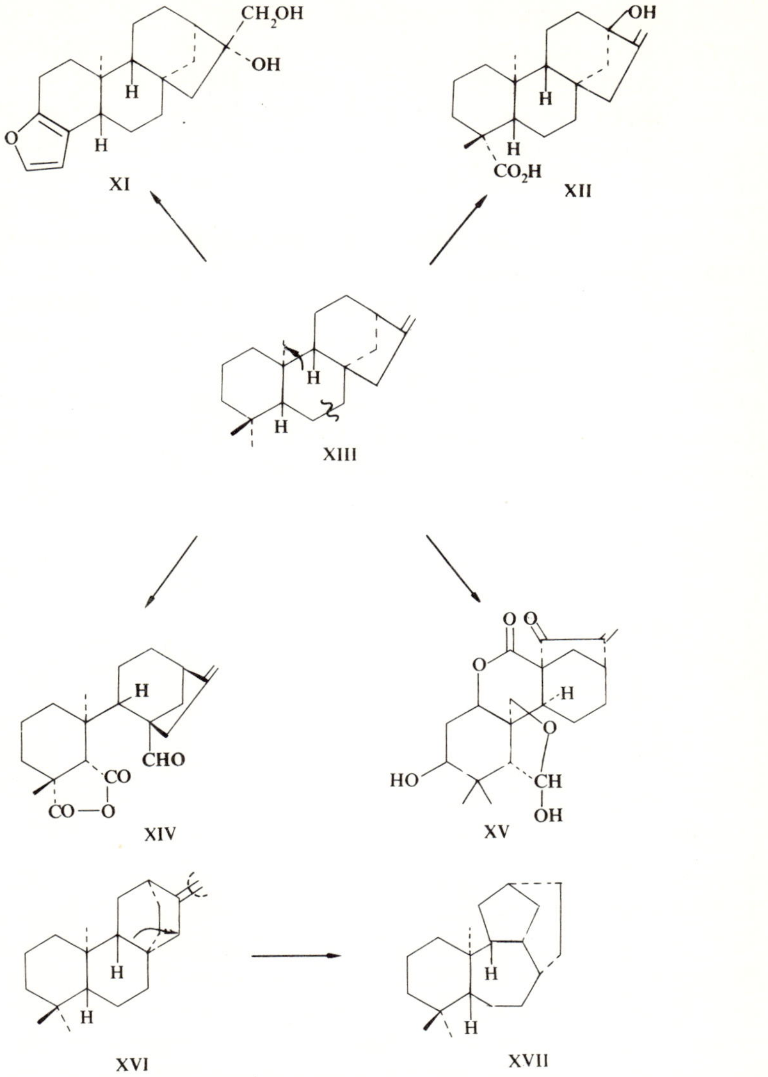

methyl and 10-carboxyl groups.[6] It is significant that only one of the geminal substituents bears the C-2 mevalonoid label—a specificity which is found elsewhere in the terpene field and contrasts with the C-10 unit of the indole alkaloids. Furthermore, this labelling pattern indicated that C-7 of the tetracyclic precursor was extruded to form the cyclopentanoid carboxylic acid of ring B. When 4R-4T-mevalonate was used[27] as a precursor, tritium was located at positions 2, 4b, and 10a, and thus these atoms are retained throughout the biosynthesis-hydroxylation at C-2 occurring with inversion.

The labelling pattern (XIX) derived[17] from (4-^{14}C)-mevalonolactone was then used to distinguish between the pinacol–pinacolone and Wagner–Meerwein mechanism for the allogibberic–gibberic acid rearrangements. In the case of the former the carbonyl group of gibberic acid should be inactive whereas in the case of the latter it should bear a label. Dehydrogenation of gibberic acid followed by oxidation gave 1, 7-dimethylfluore-

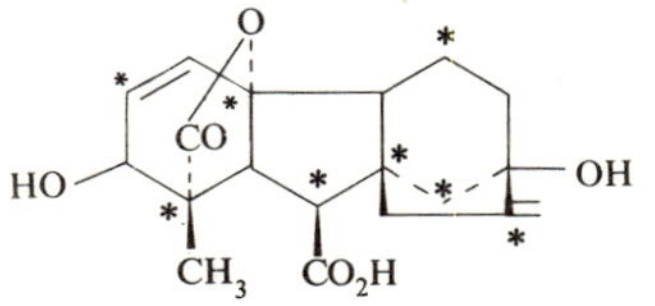

HO OH CO CH_3 CO_2H O

XVIII

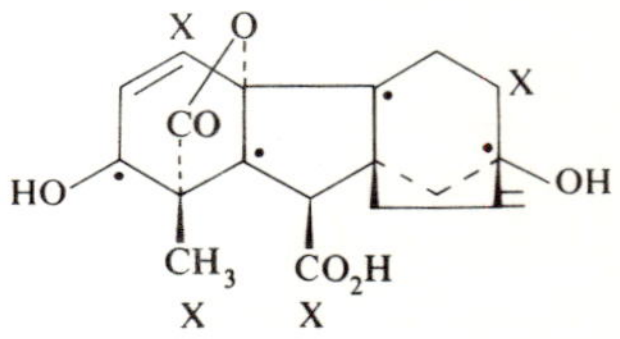

HO OH CO CH_3 CO_2H X O X X X

XIX

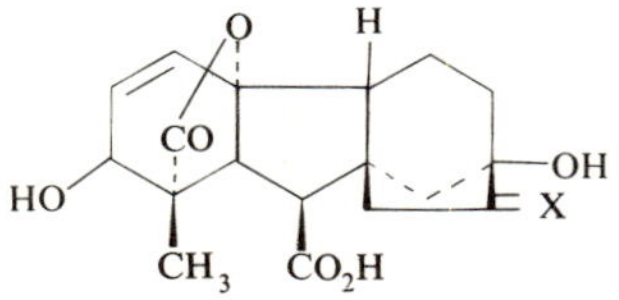

HO OH X CO CH_3 CO_2H O H

XX

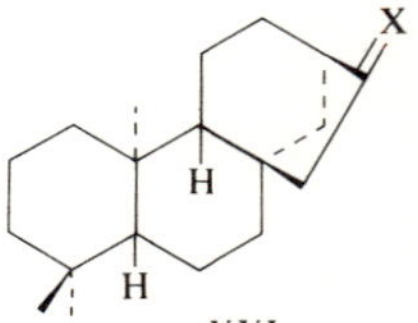

X H H

XXI

X H H $HOCH_2$ OH CO—O

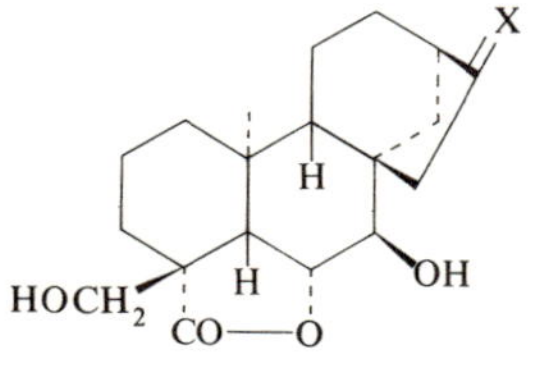

XXII

none which retained three-quarters of the activity of the parent carboxylic acid. The formation of a fluorenone which involved the loss of the D-ring bridge and also one of the labels favoured the Wagner-Meerwein mechanism. The alternative mechanism would result in retention of the four labelled atoms during dehydrogenation.

Mevalonic acid has been shown to be converted[18] to the open-chain *trans*-geranylgeranylpyrophosphate by *Echinocystis macrocarpa*. This pyrophosphate is in turn cyclized to (—)-kaurene by an enzyme system from the endosperm of immature seeds of *Echinocystis macrocarpa*.[19] A number of plant-growth retardants [e.g. 2′-isopropyl-4′-(trimethylammonium chloride)-5′-methylphenyl piperidine-1-carboxylate, Amo 1618] inhibit this stage.

The C-17-terminal methylene of the tetracyclic compounds is readily labelled by reacting the easily accessible norketones with a Wittig reagent derived from labelled methyl iodide.

Utilizing this method 17-^{14}C-(—)-kaurene (XXI) was prepared and added to the fermentation. It was specifically incorporated[21] into gibberellic acid (XX) in 5·7 per cent yield. Ozonolysis of the latter showed that 99 per cent of the activity remained in the terminal methylene group. Thus (—)-kaurene acts as precursor of gibberellic acid establishing that formation of ring D takes place prior to oxidative attack and contraction of ring B. The accompanying kauranoid metabolites, 7-hydroxy and 7, 18-dihydroxykaurenolide (XXII) were also labelled (0·05 and 0·44 per cent incorporation). (+)-Phyllocladene was not incorporated[22] into gibberellic acid. These kaurenolides were isolated[21] from a fermentation to which 2-^{14}C mevalonolactone had been added. Degradation of 7, 18-dihydroxykaurenolide established that one of the four radioactive atoms was accounted for by C-18 which was known to be β-oriented. Since (—)-kaurene acted as a common precursor to both the kaurenolides and gibberellic acid, the corresponding atom, namely the methyl group must

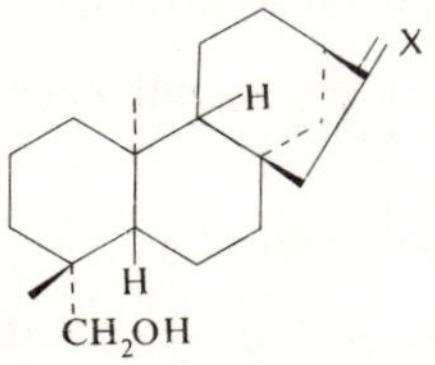

XXIII

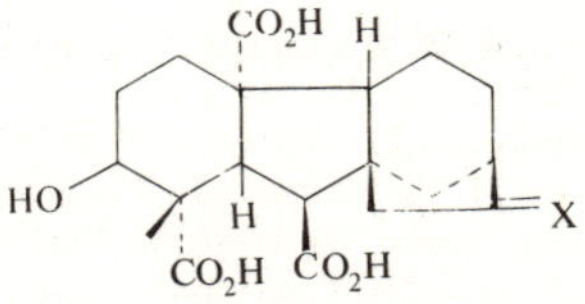

XXIV

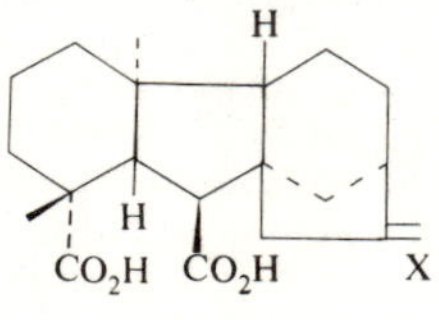

XXV

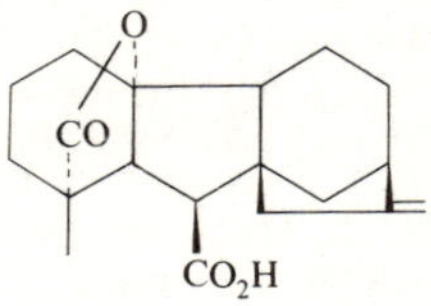

XXVI

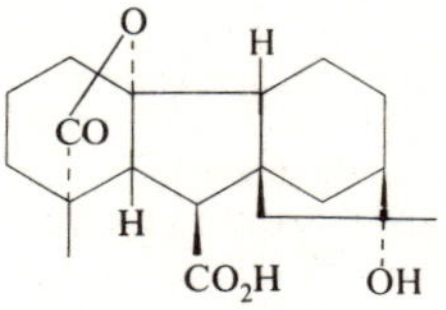

XXVII

also be β-oriented. This showed unequivocally that the lactone ring of gibberellic acid was β-oriented at a time when its orientation was in dispute. (—)-Kaurene has also been shown to be an intermediate in the biosynthesis of (—)-kaur-16-en-19-oic acid in *Echinocystis macrocarpa*.

(—)-[17-^{14}C]-Kaur-16-en-19-ol (XXIII) was added to a *Gibberella fujikuroi* fermentation.[24] Radioautography showed that gibberellin A_{13} (XXIV) and gibberellic acid were radioactive—a result which was utilized to demonstrate the stereochemistry of gibberellin A_{13}. However, [17-^{14}C]-7-hydroxykaurenolide although readily metabolized into 7, 18-dihydroxykaurenolide, did not act as a precursor of gibberellic acid. The C-20 gibberellin, gibberellin A_{12} (XXV), and its corresponding diol were incorporated[25] into gibberellic acid and gibberellin A_{13} indicating that ring-contraction takes place prior to the oxidative loss of the angular methyl group. Gibberellin A_9 (XXVI) was not incorporated into gibberellic acid, but was transformed into gibberellin A_{10} (XXVII). The sequential incorporation of mevalonic acid into (—)-kaurene and of (—)-kaurene and (—)-kaur-16-en-19-oic acid into steviol in *Stevia rebaudiana* has been described.[25]

REFERENCES

1. L. Ruzicka, *Experientia*, 9, 357 (1953).
2. E. Wenkert, *Chem. and Ind.*, 282 (1955).
3. E. Wenkert and R. Chamberlain, *J. Amer. Chem. Soc.*, **81**, 688 (1959).
4. E. Wenkert, P. W. Jeffs and J. R. Mahajan, *J. Amer. Chem. Soc.*, **86**, 2218 (1964).
5. L. H. Briggs, B. F. Cain, B. R. Davis and J. K. Wilmshurst, *Tetrahedron Letters*, **8**, 13 (1959).
6. A. J. Birch, R. W. Rickards, H. Smith, A. Harris, and W. B. Whalley, *Tetrahedron*, **7**, 241 (1959).
7. W. B. Whalley, *Tetrahedron*, **18**, 43 (1962).
8. A. I. Scott, F. McCapra, F. Comer, S. A. Sutherland, D. W. Young, G. A. Sim, and G. Ferguson, *Tetrahedron*, **20**, 1339 (1964).
9. A. H. Kapadi, R. R. Sobti and Sukh Dev, *Tetrahedron Letters*, 2729 (1965).
10. B. E. Cross, R. H. B. Galt and J. R. Hanson, *J. Chem. Soc.*, 2944 (1963).
11. C. A. Henrick and P. R. Jefferies, *Tetrahedron Letters*, 1507 (1964).
12. D. H. R. Barton, *Quart. Rev.*, **3**, 36 (1949).
13. F. E. King, T. J. King, and K. G. Neill, *J. Chem. Soc.*, 1055 (1953).
14. B. E. Cross, R. H. B. Galt and J. R. Hanson, *J. Chem. Soc.*, 295 (1964).
15. T. Kubota, T. Matsura, T. Tsutsui, S. Uyee, M. Takahashi, H. Irie, A. Numata, T. Fujita, T. Okamoto, M. Natsume, Y. Kawazoe, K. Sudo, T. Ikeda, M. Tomoeda, S. Kanatomo, T. Kosuki, and M. Adocki, *Tetrahedron*, **22**, 1659 (1966).
16. R. C. Cookson and M. E. Trevett, *J. Chem. Soc.*, 3121 (1956).
17. A. J. Birch, R. W. Rickards, H. Smith, J. Winter, and W. B. Turner, *Chem. and Ind.*, 401 (1960).
18. J. E. Graebe, D. T. Dennis, C. D. Upper and C. A. West, *J. Biol. Chem.*, **240**, 1847 (1965).
19. C. D. Upper and C. A. West, in the press.
20. D. T. Dennis, C. D. Upper and C. A. West, *Plant. Physiol.*, **40**, 945 (1965).
21. B. E. Cross, R. H. B. Galt and J. R. Hanson, *J. Chem. Soc.*, 295 (1964).
22. A. J. Birch and J. Winter, *J. Chem. Soc.*, 5547 (1963).
23. D. T. Dennis and C. A. West, in the press.
24. R. H. B. Galt, *J. Chem. Soc.*, 3143 (1965).

25. B. E. Cross and K. Norton, *Chem. Comm.*, 535 (1965); B. E. Cross, R. H. B. Galt and K. Norton, *Tetrahedron*, **24**, 231 (1968).
26. E. Wenkert and Z. Kumazawa, *Chem. Comm.*, 140 (1968); T. McCreadie and K. H. Overton, *Chem. Comm.*, 288 (1968).
27. J. R. Hanson, A. Hough and A. F. White, *Chem. Comm.*, in the press (1968).
28. R. D. Bennett, E. R. Lieber and E. Heftmann, *Phytochemistry*, **6**, 1107 (1967); J. R. Hanson and A. F. White, *Phytochemistry*, **7**, (1968), in the press.

APPENDIX

PHYSICAL CONSTANTS OF THE NATURALLY OCCURRING TETRACYCLIC DITERPENOIDS

KAURENE-PHYLLOCLADENE CLASS

Hydrocarbons		m.p.	$[\alpha]_D$	Source	Text
(−)-Kaurene	$C_{20}H_{32}$	50–50·5°	−80°	*Agathis australis* *Gibberella fujikuroi* Members of the Podocarpaceae (see text for taxonomic survey)	2.2 2.2
(+)-Kaurene	$C_{20}H_{32}$	49°	+74°	*Podocarpus ferrugineus* (see text)	2.2
(−)-Isokaurene	$C_{20}H_{32}$	64°	−26°	*Cryptomeria japonica*	2.2
(+)-Phyllocladene	$C_{20}H_{32}$	98°	+16°	*Phyllocladus rhomboidalis*	2.1
(+)-Isophyllocladene	$C_{20}H_{32}$	112°	+24°	*Cupressus macrocarpa*	2.1
(−)-Isophyllocladene	$C_{20}H_{32}$	111°	−25°	*Sciadopitys verticillata*	2.1

Alcohols		m.p.	$[\alpha]_D$	Source	Text
(−)-Kaur-16-en-3α, 19-diol	$C_{20}H_{34}O_2$	184–185°	−66°	*Beyeria leschenaultii*	2.7
16α-(−)-Kaurane-3α, 17, 19-triol	$C_{20}H_{34}O_3$	249–250°	−39°	*Beyeria leschenaultii*	2.7
(−)-Kaurane-16α, 17, 19-triol	$C_{20}H_{34}O_3$	224–226°	−38°	*Ricinocarpus stylosus*	2.7
Corymbol	$C_{20}H_{34}O_3$	282–283°	−4°	*Turbina corymbosa*	2.10
Grayanotoxins					
G. I	$C_{22}H_{36}O_7$	235°	−12°	*Leucothoe grayana* and other species of Rhododendron, Kalmia, Leucothoe and Lyonia	2.14
G. II	$C_{20}H_{32}O_5$	197°	−42°		
G. III	$C_{20}H_{34}O_6$	267–270°	−9°		
Cafestol	$C_{20}H_{28}O_3$	160–162°	−140°	*Coffea arabica*	2.10
Kahweol	$C_{20}H_{26}O_3$	88–90°	−270°	*Coffea arabica*	2.10
Abbeokutone	$C_{20}H_{32}O_3$	190–192°	−73°	*Didymosalpinx abbeokutae*	2.7
Trichokaurin	$C_{24}H_{34}O_7$	184–185°	−93°	*Isodon trichocarpus*	2.13

Acids		m.p.	$[\alpha]_D$	Source	Text
(–)-Kaur-16-en-19-oic acid	$C_{20}H_{32}O_2$	169–171, or 179–181°	–112°	*Ricinocarpus stylosus* *Gibberella fujikuroi* *Phebalium rude*	2.7
(–)-Kaur-16-en-18-oic acid	$C_{20}H_{32}O_2$	(Me ester 120–121°	–61°)	*Trachylobium verrucosum*	2.9
3β-Acetoxy-(–)-kaur-16-en-18-oic acid	$C_{22}H_{34}O_4$	(Me ester 134–136°	–70°)	*Trachylobium verrucosum*	2.9
Steviol (as the glycoside stevioside)	$C_{20}H_{30}O_3$	215°	–95°	*Stevia rebaudiana*	2.8
15β-Hydroxy-(–)-kaur-16-en-19-oic acid	$C_{20}H_{30}O_3$	209–210°	–107°	*Phebalium rude*	2.7
19-Hydroxy-16α-(–)-kauran-17-oic acid	$C_{20}H_{32}O_3$	207°	–66°	*Ricinocarpus stylosus*	2.7
1α, 19-Dihydroxy-16α-(–)-kauran-17-oic acid	$C_{20}H_{32}O_4$	259–260°	–56°	*Ricinocarpus stylosus*	2.7
19-Hydroxy-3-oxo-16α-(–)-kauran-17-oic acid	$C_{20}H_{30}O_4$	193–194°	–115°	*Beyeria* sp.	2.7
16α-(–)-Kauran-17, 19-dioic acid	$C_{20}H_{30}O_4$	271–272°	–108°	*Ricinocarpus stylosus*	2.7
Atractyligenin	$C_{19}H_{28}O_4$	189°	–146°	*Atractylis gummifiera*	2.11

Lactones		m.p.	$[\alpha]_D$	Source	Text
7-Hydroxykaurenolide	$C_{20}H_{28}O_3$	187–188°	–25°	*Gibberella fujikuroi*	2.3
7, 18-Dihydroxykaurenolide	$C_{20}H_{28}O_4$	211–214°	–37°	*Gibberella fujikuroi*	2.3
7, 16, 18-Dihydroxykaurenolide	$C_{20}H_{30}O_5$	250–255°	–	*Gibberella fujikuroi*	2.3
Enmein	$C_{20}H_{26}O_6$	308–312°	–136°	*Isodon japonicus*	2.13
				Isodon trichocarpus	2.13
Enmein 3-acetate	$C_{22}H_{28}O_7$	267–271°	–112°	*Isodon japonicus*	2.13
Isodocarpin	$C_{20}H_{26}O_5$	270–273°	–172°	*Isodon trichocarpus*	2.13
Nodosin	$C_{20}H_{26}O_6$	275–280°	–203°	*Isodon trichocarpus*	2.13
				Isodon japonicus	2.13
Isodotricin	$C_{21}H_{30}O_7$	240–245°	–114°	*Isodon trichocarpus*	2.13
Trichodonin	$C_{20}H_{30}O_7$	234–237°	+32°	*Isodon trichocarpus*	2.13
Ponicidin	$C_{20}H_{28}O_6$	238–241°	–118°	*Isodon japonicus*	2.13
Oridonin	$C_{20}H_{28}O_6$	248–250°	–46°	*Isodon trichocarpus*	2.13
				Isodon japonicus	2.13
Isodonal	$C_{22}H_{25}O_7$	245–247°	+92°	*Isodon japonicus*	2.13

Anhydrides		m.p.	$[\alpha]_D$	Source	Text
Fujenal	$C_{20}H_{26}O_4$	169–170°	–74°	*Gibberella fujikuroi*	2.12
Fujenoic acid	$C_{20}H_{26}O_5$	205–206°	–59°	*Gibberella fujikuroi*	2.12

GIBBERELLINS		m.p.	$[\alpha]_D$	Source	Text
A_1	$C_{19}H_{24}O_6$	255–258° 285°	+36°	*Gibberella fujikuroi*	3.7
A_2	$C_{19}H_{26}O_6$	235–237°	+12°	*Gibberella fujikuroi*	3.7
A_3(Gibberellic acid)	$C_{19}H_{22}O_6$	235°	+92°	*Gibberella fujikuroi*	3.1
A_4	$C_{19}H_{24}O_5$	222–255°	−3°	*Gibberella fujikuroi*	3.7
A_5	$C_{19}H_{22}O_5$	260–261°	−77°	*Phaseolus multiflorus*	3.7
A_6	$C_{19}H_{24}O_6$	205–209° 222–225°	−28°	*Phaseolus multiflorus*	3.7
A_7	$C_{19}H_{22}O_5$	169–172° 202°	20°	*Gibberella fujikuroi*	3.7
A_8	$C_{19}H_{24}O_7$	210–215°	+30°	*Phaseolus multiflorus*	3.7
A_9	$C_{19}H_{24}O_4$	208–211°	−22°	*Gibberella fujikuroi*	3.7
A_{10}	$C_{19}H_{26}O_5$	245–243°	+3°	*Gibberella fujikuroi*	3.7
A_{11}	$C_{19}H_{22}O_5$	242–244°	+11°	*Gibberella fujikuroi*	3.7
A_{12}	$C_{20}H_{28}O_4$	245–248°	–	*Gibberella fujikuroi*	3.9
A_{13}	$C_{20}H_{26}O_7$	194–196°	−48°	*Gibberella fujikuroi*	3.9
A_{14}	$C_{20}H_{28}O_5$	232–233·5°	−73°	*Gibberella fujikuroi*	3.9
A_{15}	$C_{20}H_{26}O_4$	274–276°	+5°	*Gibberella fujikuroi*	3.9
Gibberellin A_{16}	$C_{19}H_{24}O_6$	189–192°*	—	*Gibberella fujikuroi*	3.7
Gibberellin A_{17}	$C_{20}H_{26}O_7$	140–150°	—	*Phaseolus multiflorus*	3.9
Gibberellin A_{18}	$C_{20}H_{28}O_6$	240–242°	—	*Lucpinus luteus*	3.9
Gibberellin A_{19}	$C_{20}H_{26}O_6$	236–237°	—	*Phyllostachyis edulis*	3.9
Gibberellin A_{20}	$C_{19}H_{24}O_5$	181°	—	*Pharbitis nil*	3.7
Gibberellin A_{21}	$C_{19}H_{22}O_7$	244–246°	—	*Canavalia gladiata*	3.7
Gibberellin A_{22}	$C_{19}H_{22}O_6$	213–214°	—		3.7
		*Methyl ester.			

STACHENE CLASS		m.p.	$[\alpha]_D$	Source	Text
Stachene	$C_{20}H_{32}$	29·5–30°	+50°	*Erythroxylon monogynum*	4.1
(Hibaene)			−49·9°	*Thujopsis dolabrata* *Podocarpus ferrugineus*	
Stachenone	$C_{20}H_{30}O$	35·5–36°	+22°	*Spirostachys africana*	4.2
3-Hydroxystach-15-en-2-one	$C_{20}H_{30}O_2$	129°	+30°	*Spirostachys africana*	4.2
2-Hydroxystach-1, 15-dien-3-one	$C_{20}H_{25}O_2$	132°	+49°	*Spirostachys africana*	4.2
17-Hydroxystachene	$C_{20}H_{32}O$	121·5–123°	+67°	*Erythroxylon monogynum*	4.3
Monogynol	$C_{20}H_{32}O$	119°	+34°	*Erythroxylon monogynum*	4.3
Hibaene epoxide	$C_{20}H_{32}O$	74°	+16·3°	*Erythroxylon monogynum*	4.1
17, 19-Dihydroxystachene	$C_{20}H_{32}O_2$	178–179°	+41°	*Erythroxylon monogynum*	4.3
Beyerol	$C_{20}H_{32}O_3$	242–243°	+61°	*Beyeria leschenaultii*	4.4

Trachylobane Group		m.p.	$[\alpha]_D$	Source	Text
18-Hydroxytrachylobane	$C_{20}H_{32}O$	165°	−42°	*Trachylobium verrucosum*	2.15
Trachylobanic acid	$C_{20}H_{30}O_2$	[Me ester 110–112°	−41°]	*Trachylobium verrucosum*	2.15
3α-Hydroxytrachylobanic acid	$C_{20}H_{30}O_3$	[Me ester 160°	−61°]	*Trachylobium verrucosum*	2.15
3α-Acetoxytrachylobanic					
3α-Acetoxytrachylobanic acid	$C_{22}H_{32}O_4$	[Me ester 134°	−38°]	*Trachylobium verrucosum*	2.15

Atisine Class		m.p.	$[\alpha]_D$	Source	Text
Atiserene	$C_{20}H_{32}$	57–58°	−40°	*Erythroxylon monogynum*	

Diterpene Alkaloids		m.p.	$[\alpha]_D$	Source	Text
Aconine	$C_{25}H_{41}O_9N$	132°	+23°	*Aconitum napellus*	6.5
Aconitine	$C_{34}H_{47}O_{11}N$	204°	+17°	*Aconitum napellus*	6.5
Ajaconine	$C_{22}H_{33}O_3N$	172°	−119°	*Delphinium ajacis*	5.6
Atidine	$C_{22}H_{33}O_3N$	182–183°	−47°	*Aconitum heterophyllum*	5.6
Atisine	$C_{22}H_{33}O_2N$	57–60°	+28°	*Aconitum heterophyllum*	5.5
Bikhaconite	$C_{36}H_{51}O_{11}N$	163–164°	+16°	*Aconitum spicatum*	6.7
Browniine	$C_{25}H_{41}O_7N$	212°	+25°	*Delphinium brownii* *Delphinium cardinale*	6.4
Chasmaconitine	$C_{34}H_{47}O_9N$	181–182°	+10°	*Aconitum chasmanthum*	6.8
Chasmanine	$C_{25}H_{41}O_6N$	90–91°	+24°	*Aconitum chasmanthum*	6.8
Chasmanthinine	$C_{36}H_{49}O_9N$	160–161°	+10°	*Aconitum chasmanthum* *Delphinium confusum*	6.8
Condelphine	$C_{25}H_{39}O_6N$	156–158°	+27°	*Delphinium denudatum*	6.9
Cuauchichicine	$C_{22}H_{33}O_2N$	152–155°	−71°	*Garrya laurifolia*	5.3
Delatine	$C_{19}H_{25}O_3N$	148°	+13·5°	*Delphinium elatum*	5.9
Delavaconine	$C_{23}H_{37}O_5N$	150°	−53° (Tri Ac.)	*Aconitum* sp.	–
Delcosine	$C_{24}H_{39}O_7N$	203°	+57°	*Delphinium consolida* *Delphinium ajacis*	6.3
Delphatine	$C_{27}H_{45}O_7N$	101–106°	+39°	*Delphinium biternatum*	–
Delphelatine	$C_{30}H_{47}O_9N$	188–189°	−27°	*Delphinium elatum*	–
Delpheline	$C_{25}H_{39}O_6N$	227°	−26°	*Delphinium elatum*	6.2
Delphinine	$C_{33}H_{45}O_9N$	198–200°	+25°	*Delphinium staphisagria*	6.10
Delphonine	$C_{24}H_{39}O_7N$	78 °	+38°	*Delphinium* sp.	6.10
Delsoline	$C_{25}H_{41}O_7N$	213–216°	+52°	*Delphinium consolida*	6.3
Deltaline	$C_{27}H_{41}O_8N$	193–195°	−27°	*Delphinium barbeyi* *Delphinium occidentale* *Delphinium elatum*	–
Denudatine	$C_{21}H_{33}O_2N$	248–249°	+0·15	*Delphinium* sp.	–
Garryfoline	$C_{22}H_{33}O_2N$	130–133°	−60°	*Garrya laurifolia*	5.3
Garryine	$C_{22}H_{33}O_2N$	75–80°	−84°	*Garrya* sp.	5.2
Heteratisine	$C_{22}H_{33}O_5N$	262–267°	+40°	*Aconitum heterophyllum*	6.11
Hetisine	$C_{20}H_{27}O_3N$	253–256°	+14°	*Aconitum heterophyllum*	5.9
Hypoignavine	$C_{27}H_{31}O_5N$	239–241°	–	*Aconitum sanyoense*	5.7
Ignavine	$C_{27}H_{31}O_6N$	172–174°	+86°	*Aconitum japonicum* *Aconitum sanyoense* *Aconitum tasiromontanum*	5.7

DITERPENE ALKALOIDS		m.p.	$[\alpha]_D$	Source	Text
Indaconitine	$C_{34}H_{47}O_{10}N$	202–203°	+18°	*Aconitum chasmanthum*	6.6
Isotalatizidine	$C_{23}H_{37}O_5N$	116–117°	–	*Aconitum talissicum*	6.9
Jesaconitine	$C_{35}H_{27}O_2N$	128–131°	–17°	*Aconitum napellus*	6.5
Kobusine	$C_{20}H_{27}O_2N$	268°	+84°	*Aconitum sachalinense*	5.9
				Aconitum yesoensis	
Lycoctonine	$C_{25}H_{41}O_7N$	151–153°	+50°	*Aconitum* sp.	6.1
Mesaconitine	$C_{33}H_{45}O_{11}N$	208–209°	+26°	*Aconitum sacchalinense*	6.5
Methyl lycaconitine	$C_{37}H_{48}O_{10}N$	128°	+49°	*Delphinium elatum*	6.2
Napelline	$C_{22}H_{33}O_3N$	166°	–43°	*Aconitum napellus*	5.4
Pseudoaconitine	$C_{36}H_{51}O_{12}N$	214°	+17°	*Aconitum deinorrhizum*	6.6
				Aconitum napellus	
				Aconitum spicatus	
Songorine	$C_{22}H_{31}O_3N$	212°	–	*Aconitum napellus*	5.4
Talatizidine	$C_{23}H_{37}O_5N$	218–219°	–20°	*Aconitum talissicum*	6.9
Veatchine	$C_{22}H_{33}O_2N$	119–120°	–69°	*Garrya* sp.	5.2

INDEX

OTHER TITLES IN THE SERIES IN ORGANIC CHEMISTRY

Vol. 1. WATERS—*Vistas in Free-radical Chemistry*
Vol. 2. TOPCHIEV *et al.*—*Boron Fluoride and its Compounds as Catalysts in Organic Chemistry*
Vol. 3. JANSSEN—*Synthetic Analgesics—Part I: Diphenylpropylamines*
Vol. 4. WILLIAMS—*Homolytic Aromatic Substitution*
Vol. 5. JACKMAN—*Applications of Nuclear Magnetic Resonance Spectroscopy in Organic Chemistry*
Vol. 6. GEFTER—*Organophosphorus Monomers and Polymers*
Vol. 7. SCOTT—*Interpretations of the Ultraviolet Spectra of Natural Products*
Vol. 8. HELLERBACH *et al.*—*Synthetic Analgesics—Part II: (A) Morphinans. (B) 6,7-Benzomorphans*